T0075141

NAVIGATING THE ICU

A GUIDE FOR PATIENTS AND FAMILIES

By Alex Gottsch, MHS, MSN, RN

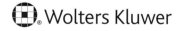. Wolters Kluwer

Philadelphia • Baltimore • New York • London
Buenos Aires • Hong Kong • Sydney • Tokyo

Acquisitions Editor: Keith Donnellan
Development Editor: Ariel S. Winter
Production Project Manager: Kirstin Johnson
Marketing Manager: Kirsten Watrud
Manager, Graphic Arts & Design: Stephen Druding
Manufacturing Coordinator: Beth Welsh
Prepress Vendor: TNQ Technologies

Copyright © 2023 Wolters Kluwer.

All rights reserved. This book is protected by copyright. No part of this book may be reproduced or transmitted in any form or by any means, including as photocopies or scanned-in or other electronic copies, or utilized by any information storage and retrieval system without written permission from the copyright owner, except for brief quotations embodied in critical articles and reviews. Materials appearing in this book prepared by individuals as part of their official duties as U.S. government employees are not covered by the above-mentioned copyright. To request permission, please contact Wolters Kluwer at Two Commerce Square, 2001 Market Street, Philadelphia, PA 19103, via email at permissions@lww.com, or via our website at shop.lww.com (products and services).

9 8 7 6 5 4 3 2 1

Printed in Singapore

Library of Congress Cataloging-in-Publication Data

ISBN-13: 978-1-975191-38-2

Cataloging in Publication data available on request from publisher.

This work is provided "as is," and the publisher disclaims any and all warranties, express or implied, including any warranties as to accuracy, comprehensiveness, or currency of the content of this work.

This work is no substitute for individual patient assessment based upon healthcare professionals' examination of each patient and consideration of, among other things, age, weight, gender, current or prior medical conditions, medication history, laboratory data and other factors unique to the patient. The publisher does not provide medical advice or guidance and this work is merely a reference tool. Healthcare professionals, and not the publisher, are solely responsible for the use of this work including all medical judgments and for any resulting diagnosis and treatments.

Given continuous, rapid advances in medical science and health information, independent professional verification of medical diagnoses, indications, appropriate pharmaceutical selections and dosages, and treatment options should be made and healthcare professionals should consult a variety of sources. When prescribing medication, healthcare professionals are advised to consult the product information sheet (the manufacturer's package insert) accompanying each drug to verify, among other things, conditions of use, warnings and side effects and identify any changes in dosage schedule or contraindications, particularly if the medication to be administered is new, infrequently used or has a narrow therapeutic range. To the maximum extent permitted under applicable law, no responsibility is assumed by the publisher for any injury and/or damage to persons or property, as a matter of products liability, negligence law or otherwise, or from any reference to or use by any person of this work.

shop.lww.com

MKO522

*Dedicated to the Patients and Their Families
Suffering from Coronavirus in the ICU*

Foreword

The intensive care unit (ICU) provides highly specialized and life-saving treatments. Admission to the ICU is often sudden, and the life-threatening aspects of care and antecedent events are daunting for patients, their families, and health professionals alike. The COVID-19 pandemic has pulled back the curtains, underscoring the intensity, complexity, and emotion of the intensive care environment. But these are not new circumstances; the literature is replete in these descriptions of the challenges of the environment and emphasizing the need for communication and support of patients and their families.

In this text, *Navigating the ICU: A Guide for Patients and Families*, Alex Gottsch, through the eyes of an experienced ICU nurse, provides a succinct and informative description of the ICU environment, roles and responsibilities of key personnel, potential events, and demystifies steps in the ICU journey. The goal of this book is to make the ICU experience less overwhelming and families feel they are included in the medical team. The book is well organized in clear and succinct chapters, allowing family members to dip in and out of key information sources to assist in navigating the ICU during this stressful time. I can also see this as a resource for ICU survivors who seek to piece together the elements of what is often a confusing and daunting experience.

Understanding the role of the ICU, the work, rhythm of life, and activities from the perspective of a nurse is empowering and should be comforting to families. As the most trusted profession, and in the ICU, highly skilled practitioners, nurses take care of patients every minute of the day and are literally watching every breath and counting every heart beat to ensure patients are safe and taken care of.

For the families who have the need to pick up this book, I hold you in my thoughts and prayers. Seeing a loved one in the ICU is a truly scary and daunting experience. Use this text to help you feel more involved in your loved one's care. Effective communication is critical and sometimes asking the right questions is important in getting the information you need. Reach out to the nurses—they are there to support you—and take the time to understand the roles of different professionals in the healthcare team.

During this time it is also important to take care of yourself. Taking time to eat, sleep, and exercise can sustain you in this challenging time. Reach out and ask for help; people are ready, willing, and able to assist you and your family. This text will help you; it will provide you with information that will make you feel more in control of this often overwhelming situation.

I wish you all the very best at this challenging time and hope for peace and comfort for you and your family.

Patricia M. Davidson, RN, PhD, FAAN
Dean and Professor
Johns Hopkins School of Nursing

Introduction

The need for this book became painfully clear as COVID-19 swept through our country.

Infected people needed life-saving medical care. Hospitals overflowed as the virus spread. Constant alarms, emergencies, and deaths were exhausting. Each new surge required more from medical staff already spread thin. ICU care, stressful without a pandemic, became even more demanding.

Communication, a critical part of hospital care, suffered.

With or without COVID-19, communication in the ICU is always hard. In this high-stress environment, many people work together to quickly treat the sickest patients, often with distraught families looking for answers no one knows. Communication stalls as the ICU team focuses on treatments, the patient endures therapies, and the family tries to not interrupt. As a result, families think they are excluded, patients feel isolated, and the ICU team hopes their best care is the right care. However, when done well, communication supports everyone involved.

Although nothing can be guaranteed, the best experience is most likely when the patient, family, and ICU team are in sync. When this happens, patients have an understanding of their health and where it is heading. They have support from their family by their side, and the ICU team works seamlessly with them to develop and deliver an agreed-upon plan for care. Everyone feels like they have been informed, advised, and heard. Of course, people die. But in those times, people die with loved ones close, saying goodbye, and cherishing those last moments.

COVID-19 makes times like those nearly impossible.

Patients with COVID-19 are isolated all day, every day. Families cannot be by their side without fear of spreading the infection. The patient's most common human interactions consist of phone or video calls with family, and medical personnel who are dressed from head to toe in protective equipment.

Usually, these patients are receiving oxygen. Small movements exhaust them as they struggle for each breath. Eating is a terrible and sometimes impossible chore as they have to time each swallow between labored and rapid breaths. Proning (laying on the stomach) can buy patients time, but eating more than a few bites in this position—when breathing alone is tiring—rarely happens. Face down in bed, starving, and struggling to get enough air, is how many COVID-19 patients spend their days. Throughout this time, questions flood their minds: How long will this last? Will they be able to save me? Will I see my family again?

Although great advances have been made, there is no cure for COVID-19. Instead, ICU teams have to try imperfect remedies, unsure of how patients will recover. All reasonable options are on the table, but none provide a definitive remedy.

The lungs are COVID-19's main target, but it can affect all parts of the body, with the kidneys, heart, and brain also receiving the worst of the virus's impact. Intubation—inserting a tube to help the patient breathe—can save patients with other lung diseases, but the same does not always hold true with this infection. The kidneys hopefully will survive, but will dialysis be needed? Can the heart withstand the immune system's overreaction aimed at combating the infection? Will there be any lasting brain injury?

It can take weeks for COVID-19 patients to recover and leave the hospital. Unfortunately, more time is usually needed to regrow muscle and heal mental and physical scars after the hospital stay. Destroyed lung tissue can take years to heal. For many of these patients, a life dependent on oxygen or a lung transplant linger as the only options.

Waiting outside, the family prays for good news, searching for any sign that today was better than yesterday. When meeting with the ICU team, complex medical topics are explained that are difficult to learn, even when without stress.

Countless times, the family receives a call in the middle of the night. Changing vital signs, statistics, and medical procedures are hastily described with the best intentions. Quickly, a literal life or death decision has to be made. Inevitably, the overwhelmed relative asks for more time to decide and is told that there is none. Their loved one is on the brink of death, and action is needed to save their life.

Panic, stress, and fear fill the voices of the family members agreeing to another procedure. Faced with what seems to be no choice, the family, speaking on behalf of the now-incapacitated patient, chooses anything that glimmers of hope. Did they understand the risks? Did they do what the patient would have wanted? Was that the right decision?

Too often, both the patient and family never get to say goodbye, because they did not realize the path the infection was going to take as the ambulance pulled away. The breathing tube was inserted not long afterward, the patient now cannot respond, and it is time to say goodbye forever. The worst times are made worse by having to say everything you wanted to say earlier through a video call.

As an ICU nurse caring for patients with COVID-19, I noticed the toll communication breakdowns were taking in the ICU. Communication, compassion, and delivering the right care that aligns with the patient's wishes became more difficult during the pandemic. COVID-19 widened the gaps in communication between patients, families, and the ICU staff. However, these gaps were always looming, even for the most united relationships.

This COVID-19 realization made clear the need for all patients, with any illness, and their families to fully understand what occurs in the ICU. In an environment where a positive outcome cannot be promised, where there are risks to everything, and where even the most stable patient can become unstable in an instant, an effective partnership between patients, families, and the ICU team is vital.

Unfortunately, the best plan for treatment is often unclear to the patient, family, or ICU team. When this happens, decisions can be made that do not best serve the patient. Sometimes a strong-willed family pushes a reluctant patient to go forward with an operation that the ICU team thinks is hopeless. I have also seen family members change an unresponsive patient's last wish and insist upon prolonged life support, forcing that patient to a bedbound life that was explicitly rejected. Even the ICU team may recommend care that the patient or family simply does not want.

Whether these moments are in the peak surge of a COVID-19 ICU or any time in other ICUs, communication too often is lost. Too often, patients and families feel as if there is no other choice. No choice but to abandon control. No choice but to go full speed ahead. No real choice as decisions need to be made quickly in a technical language the family is just barely grasping, in an unfamiliar environment echoing with alarms, with their loved one, ridden with tubes and supported by machines, on the verge of death.

Yet there is an important choice. Families can choose to be not just a passive observer but an active participant. Choose to become familiar with the environment, understand the machines, and learn the language. Choose to partner with the ICU team as another, well-informed advocate for the patient. In every ICU, when the family feels empowered and is involved in care, the experience for everyone, especially the patient, is better.

This book will help you. It will guide you through the ICU experience. As a nurse, I spend every day explaining in detail—and in plain language—the entire care a patient is receiving, so the patient, family, and ICU team are on the same page. In this book, I describe important concepts to know, the right questions to ask, and what the best care looks like. I clearly explain the medical procedures, machines, tests, and other subjects that occur daily in every ICU. I also explain important actions to take now to improve recovery inside the hospital and after leaving. This book will empower you to make the right decisions. Use this book to join the ICU team, to enable the best care possible, and to give the patient the best chance at recovery.

How This Book Helps Patients and Families

The ICU can be a scary place. It is stressful even thinking about a loved one needing the care that an ICU provides. The medical jargon, the pressure to make stressful decisions quickly, the intrusion of unfamiliar people into personal space, and wondering whether life will ever be the same are all upsetting. A predictable outcome is rarely foreseeable, and complications are always a possibility. Understandably, patients and families often are underprepared and overwhelmed when they find themselves in an ICU.

This guide is for those in the ICU who are receiving care or are supporting a loved one. As an ICU nurse, I have cared for many patients over the years. I have worked in all the adult ICUs at Duke Hospital and have traveled throughout the country working at other hospitals, learning which practices are best for patients and what matters most to them. This book will explain who the medical personnel are, what they do, and why they are important for recovery. It will clearly explain the common procedures, how each affects patients, and mention details and tips that are helpful for patients and family members. This book covers important components of ICU care and helps patients and families feel comfortable interacting with the ICU team. Readers will be enabled to help ensure that care provided is safe, effective, and achieving the goals of the patient. Overall, my hope is this book will make the experience less overwhelming and help patients and their families feel included in the ICU team—which they are! It will identify what needs to be known and how to navigate the ICU during this stressful time. Many have been there before, and many have fully recovered.

Please note that when "family" is written, this can also mean support persons who the patient wants included in their care. So, this can mean literal family or other people who the patient trusts. Additionally, some of my suggestions are directed at family or support persons. However, these suggestions may be important for patients as well. As always, the ICU team can provide help in any situation.

How to Use This Book

In an attempt to explain everything of importance to all ICU patients, this book may repeat a common issue in communication: giving too much information at one time. Some patients and their families prefer short explanations as they process the recent events.

So, everyone may not need the amount of detail provided in this book. Also, each patient will not experience everything in this guide. Therefore, a way to learn about something while avoiding too much information is to use the index. When something occurs or a procedure is suggested, look it up in the back of the book. Of course, the table of contents also gives readers a guide for what may interest them.

However, there are a few sections that everyone should read, because they cover important topics for every ICU patient. These are listed as follows:

- Chapter 1—The Staff
- Chapter 2—A Typical Day
- Chapter 3—The Basics
- *Informed Consent* in Chapter 4
- *Medication Timing* in Chapter 5
- *Delirium* in Chapter 7
- Chapter 9—Essentials for the ICU Patient
- Chapter 10—How to Help the Patient During Downtime
- Chapter 11—How to Prepare Now for a Better Life After Hospitalization
- Chapter 12—Where the Patient Recovers After the Hospital
- Chapter 14—Critical Questions That Determine the Right Care

Throughout the book there are "Nurse's Notes." These mention important tips and considerations that can make a difference for the patient and family. Additionally, there is a glossary at the end to help understand medical terms. The website, NavigatingTheICU. com, contains extra material and links to all the resources mentioned throughout the book.

Most importantly, this guide should be used alongside the medical personnel. They will be able to answer any remaining questions and provide further resources. Patient recovery takes a team effort, so everyone has to work together to give the patient the best chance.

Acknowledgments

Thanks to my family and friends for your love and support. A special thanks to those who helped make this guide better. I appreciate you.

Contents

15 Important Topics When Discussing
the End of the Patient's Life 149

1

The Staff

The introduction to the intensive care unit (ICU) begins with those working there every day. Although people are familiar with the traditional roles, such as a doctor or nurse, many other staff contribute to the patient's recovery. Each one of them is a crucial part of the medical team that is vital to providing thorough patient care.

The ICU staff members that make up this team and their roles are described below.

The Nurses

The patient and family spend the most time with the bedside nurses. Their first job is to care for the patient.

From providing such fundamental human needs as feeding and bathing, to coordinating care across the hospital system, the nurses manage the care that a patient receives. The nurses administer medications, monitor their patients for signs of bettering or worsening health, and ensure the prescribed treatments and procedures occur.

Nurses also are a great resource for patients and families because they are accessible and can contact all of the healthcare team members. In most ICUs, the nurse will have one or two patients. This allows for continuous monitoring of the patient and a swift reaction to a patient's needs. Because changes occur quickly in critically ill patients, the nurse must be able to respond rapidly to any crisis.

An additional nurse, the supervising <u>charge nurse</u>, assists all of the nurses. The charge nurse organizes the flow of patients and personnel within the ICU, such as transferring patients and assigning nurses to patients for the next shift. Although a great source of information regarding unit policies and workflow, the charge nurse may not be as familiar with the patient as the bedside nurse.

Nurse's Note

☐ If you like your current nurse and would prefer them for future shifts, you can request this from the charge nurse.

Figure 1.1   The Nursing Ladder

This diagram shows the general hierarchy of nurses in the hospital. If the bedside nurse cannot solve a problem, the charge nurse may be better suited, followed by the nursing manager, etc. The nursing director or chief nursing officer is the lead nurse in the organization.

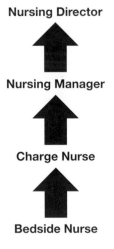

Nursing Director

Nursing Manager

Charge Nurse

Bedside Nurse

The Doctors

The plan for a patient's care usually is directed by the doctors, or physicians. Many different doctors work together to treat a patient. This group can be called the ICU team, primary team, or main team. Doctors who are trained in treating patients in the ICU may be called intensivists. This team usually consists of the attending, fellow, resident, and intern.

The head decision-maker at any point of the treatment is the <u>attending</u> physician. The attending is the most senior, has the most experience caring for patients in the ICU, will direct the patient's overall plan of care, and bears ultimate responsibility for the medical team. Attending physicians are considered to have finished their training in their specialty. There are many specialties, such as cardiology, neurology, anesthesiology, etc.

If the hospital trains doctors (known as a teaching hospital), the next-highest decision-maker is the <u>fellow</u>. This doctor, although very experienced, is still considered to be learning from the attending in their specialty. This training can last from 1 to 3 years.

Learning from both the attending and fellow are the <u>residents</u>, who are in training for 3 to 7 years, depending on their specialty. Most of a patient's experience with the doctors is with residents. They are expected to know the current health data of the patients at all times. Residents who are in their first year may be called interns. They have just graduated from medical school and are not yet allowed to practice medicine by themselves.

Figure 1.2 The Doctor Ladder

This diagram shows the general hierarchy of doctors in a teaching hospital. If the intern cannot solve a problem, the resident may be better suited, followed by the fellow, etc. The medical director or chief medical officer is the lead doctor of the organization.

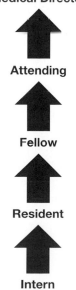

Medical Director

Attending

Fellow

Resident

Intern

If the ICU team is not expertly trained in a part of the body involved in the illness, such as the kidneys, brain, heart, or blood infection, they will consult those who are. Typically, these consultants, or specialists, are other doctors who are experts in that part of the body. They will assess the patient regularly and give the ICU team recommendations. There are times when different specialists will make conflicting recommendations. The ICU team decides which path to take, as they are most familiar with the patient.

Nurse's Note

- Because many doctors interact with the patient, it can be confusing to determine who is part of which team. You can always ask who they are, how long they will be assigned to the patient, and what their specialty is.
- Doctors fall under the category of provider, meaning they identify the illness, prescribe therapies, and determine the patient's medical plan.

The Nurse Practitioners and Physician Assistants

Nurse practitioners (NPs) and physician assistants (PAs) are other types of providers. They are also referred to as advanced practice providers (APPs). NPs and PAs have graduate school training in medicine. They help manage the patient's medical care and work closely with the doctors. Depending on where they work, they also may be able to provide care and perform procedures without the guidance of an attending doctor.

The Respiratory Therapists

Working closely with the nurses, physicians, and other healthcare providers are the respiratory therapists (RTs). They are experts in all things related to breathing. The RTs assist all patients who need oxygen, from the small amount provided by the nasal cannula, up to the total support of the breathing machine. The nurse knows how to work this equipment, but the RTs are experts. The RTs may also administer breathing treatments and assist with lung-related procedures.

The Pharmacists

The <u>pharmacist</u> is another important part of the ICU team. The pharmacists double-check and approve all medications and dosages that are prescribed. They make sure the patient's medications are having the desired effect while avoiding unwanted interactions between medications. Furthermore, they monitor important medication levels in the blood to make sure they are in safe ranges.

The Physical and Occupational Therapists

To return to their life, the patient needs to have strength and coordination. Everyone loses muscle while recovering in the ICU. The resulting weakness makes it harder to safely accomplish everyday activities. These are called activities of daily living (ADLs), which include bathing, dressing, feeding, toileting, and moving around in the environment. The <u>physical therapist</u> (PT) helps the patients to regain the strength to move within their environment, and the <u>occupational therapist</u> (OT) helps the patients practice those ADLs. In some cases, these therapists may come daily, and they may leave homework for the patient. Physical and occupational therapy are essential to getting out of the hospital and remaining healthy.

The Speech-Language Pathologists

The <u>speech-language pathologist</u> (SLP), or speech therapist, helps patients who have trouble with eating, drinking, or speaking. For instance, a stroke patient with facial weakness will need help from the SLP to eat without risking choking. The SLP may have to see if the patient can safely swallow before they are allowed to eat or drink. The SLP can recommend types of food that are safest for the patient, as well as tips for eating, drinking, and taking medicine. Additionally, the SLP can help patients strengthen their voice and ability to speak. For instance, a stroke patient may have trouble speaking, and the SLP can help improve their ability to communicate.

The Social Workers and Case Managers

Social workers and case managers are essential in coordinating the patient's needs in the hospital and navigating options when they leave. They help the patient and family access available social services, such as financial, disability, rehabilitation, counseling, support networks, etc. They will evaluate the patient's short- and long-term goals and follow up to make sure they are met.

Social workers and case managers also work with insurance companies to connect patients to organizations outside of the hospital, such as long-term care, rehabilitation, home health, hospice, etc. They can also provide paperwork needed to explain why patients missed work, to file disability claims, etc. These ICU representatives play a critical role in empowering patients to stay out of the hospital after discharge.

The Ethics Committee/Ethicists

Sometimes, the best plan for the patient may not be agreed upon by everyone. It is best when patients, their family, and their medical team are united on a path forward. This can be difficult during hard times. Separate from the ICU team, the ethics committee is very helpful in making sense of complicated situations and providing guidance about what may be important moving forward. If necessary, the ICU team knows how to contact them so they can help shed light on challenging scenarios.

The Nurse Aides

The value of the nurse aides, medical assistants, and patient care technicians is huge. Sometimes referred to as techs, they help the unit run smoothly by assisting in many things, such as testing blood sugar levels, helping a patient eat, repositioning a patient, stocking rooms, etc. They are usually very busy because their services are needed throughout the unit.

Other Vital Staff Who May Be Regularly Seen in the ICU

- Chaplains and spiritual services are valuable for many patients. They provide spiritual care for all denominations, even if the patient is not in distress. They also offer support for families, atheists, and those who do not identify with any religion.
- Dieticians optimize nutrition for patients.
- Mobility technicians are experts in the important task of movement. They assist patients in moving so they avoid the many negative consequences of being stationary.

2

A Typical Day

Although the intensive care unit (ICU) is fully staffed at all times, there is a rhythm to the unit that is essential to know. Depending on the time and day, members of the ICU team are more readily available for questions and concerns. Those who learn the schedule can best take advantage of the available resources. There are times when it is important to be present and times when the family can focus on other priorities.

Activity in the ICU mirrors the flow of regular life. Days tend to be busier than nights, and weekends and holidays can be slower than weekdays. Of course, ICU staff are prepared for anything at any time, but it is during the day on weekdays that the most personnel are available for procedures and guiding patient care.

The Most Important Part of the Day to Be at the Bedside

The most important moment in the day occurs during <u>rounds</u>. This usually begins in the morning around 8:00 AM. The whole medical team, including the doctors, pharmacist, respiratory therapist, dietician, and nurse, comes to the patient's room. The patient's entire course of illness is discussed. The medical team explains what has been done for the patient, what the current issues are, and what the plan is for treatment. This usually is when the providers decide if it safe to transfer the patient out of the ICU.

After rounds, the team is working on all of the patients in the ICU at the same time, so decisions can be delayed. The morning rounds are when everyone is focused on the patient. Therefore, this is the best time for family members to interact with the medical team, get updated with the latest information, and ask the most important questions.

Nurse's Note

- The timing of rounds can be unpredictable. Rounds can be delayed because emergencies need to be addressed, and the team discusses each patient in detail. Because of this, it is best to set aside the entire morning. As your time in the ICU grows, the different members of the team, their schedules, and the rhythm of the unit will become familiar.

- Ask the nurse when the morning rounds usually are and mention any current questions you may have.

- Write down your questions and concerns before rounds so that you don't forget them. A lot of information is presented quickly, so it helps to have everything in front of you.

- If your hospital does not round, or all of your questions cannot be answered during rounding, you can ask the nurse to have the doctor update you on the plan at some point during the day.

- Please see Appendix 1 for a guide to use during rounds (page 163).

The Schedule for the Day

Although every hospital is different, they all follow a similar schedule. Mornings tend to be busy, with rounds and breakfast occurring around 8:00 AM. Most of the medications are given during that time. Lunch occurs around noon. The physical therapist, occupational therapist, and speech therapist visit in the morning or afternoon. Typically, transfers to other floors occur in the afternoon, but they can happen at any time. Dinner comes around 6:00 PM. Unfortunately, it is hard for patients to sleep through the night because they need to be closely monitored. The busy times during the night are 8:00 PM, midnight, and 4:00 AM.

Nurse's Note

- Some hospitals build quiet time into their days and nights. For instance, 2:00 to 4:00 AM and 2:00 to 4:00 PM may be reserved for resting.
- Procedures occur as needed, at any time during the day or night.

The Staff Shift Change

Each hospital is different, but many follow the same routine. The attending physicians tend to work 1 full week where they are available at all times. Some hospitals have their fellows, residents, nurse practitioners, or physician assistants working 12- to 24-hour days, so their schedules will vary. Nurses tend to work three 12-hour shifts per week. These shifts usually change at 7:00 AM and 7:00 PM.

During the change of shift, the staff who are completing their shift will give those who are starting their shift a detailed assessment of the patient. Referred to as the report, it is vital to the care of the patient and should not be interrupted. They describe the patient's history, the current issues, and the plan.

3

The Basics

This chapter presents some common aspects of the intensive care unit (ICU) that are experienced by many patients and families.

Why the ICU

A common question is "Why am I (or my loved one) in the ICU?" There are many reasons why a patient may be admitted to an ICU, and they all have the same underlying factors: the need to constantly monitor the patient and be able to provide maximum medical support. Typically, without some medicine, machine, or intervention, these patients will not survive.

Patients in the ICU are very sick or have the potential to need lifesaving care. A provider is available at all hours, and nurses have at most two patients, who are continuously monitored. Basically, the patient and their vital signs are watched at all times. Some patients or family members are confused about why they are in the ICU yet do not "seem" sick. Usually, the ICU staff has been busy stabilizing the patient with medical care. Or the staff is watching them closely, because the patient could quickly deteriorate and require immediate, emergency interventions. In these situations, it is important that the ICU personnel and equipment spring into action as quickly as possible. Practicing rapid and lifesaving medicine is why the ICU exists.

Admission Into the ICU

Typically, a patient can be transferred to the ICU in three ways. One way is through the emergency department (ED), where providers, nurses, and staff have been helping the patient. The ED team determines if the patient needs ICU-level care, and the ICU team accepts the patient. Depending on the patient's illness and available bed space within the hospital, this process may take hours. Once an ICU room opens, the patient is taken there.

The second way a patient arrives in the ICU is from what is called a Rapid Response. If a patient in a different unit is getting worse, the nurse calls for a Rapid Response Team to examine the patient. This team is familiar with the symptoms that need ICU-level care. Some of these are a need for more oxygen, low blood pressure, rapid breathing, or not being able to stay awake. If ICU-level care is needed, they will transfer the patient there.

Another common route to the ICU is after surgery. For high-risk operations, patients need to have the supervision provided by the ICU in case of any complications. Typically, the patient, family, and medical team will plan to have the patient recover in the ICU. After surgery, the patient is brought to their room by the operative team and postoperative care is coordinated in the ICU.

However the admission occurs, the patient and family are exhausted, and the ICU is likely an unfamiliar environment. This time is filled with a mixture of anxiety and relief, answers and resulting questions, and activity and stillness. Usually, the patient is brought into the room, while the family is asked to stay outside or in the waiting room. This is to allow more room for the ICU staff to examine the patient, conduct any procedures, and attach the monitoring devices. Each patient may be tested for some common infections, such as MRSA (a.k.a. staph). After admission, family may be allowed to stay with the patient depending on the hospital's policies. Just in case, ask what the visitation policy is. From this point, a plan will be made for the patient's treatment, and the patient will be monitored continuously.

Nurse's Note

- A welcome packet may be provided in the patient's room with helpful orientation information. Ask the nurse or unit secretary for one if it is not there.

- Ask the nurse if a password is needed to get updates on the patient when calling. This is used to protect patient privacy.

- Please let the staff know if the patient has any dietary, cultural, or spiritual requests. The team wants to treat you the way you want to be treated.

Monitoring the Patient

A monitoring device is always attached to the patient. At a minimum, this is reading the patient's blood pressure, heartbeats per minute (heart rate), breaths per minute (respiratory rate), and percentage of oxygen in the blood, all known as <u>vital signs</u>. How these measurements are taken can be seen by following the cords from the monitor down to the patient. The nurse tries to position the wires so they are out of the patient's way.

High and low limits are set for each vital sign, and the monitor alarms if one goes above or below that limit. Alarms save lives. They are also a common annoyance. Often the monitor will alarm for minor reasons, such as a repositioning patient or a detached cord.

Although many alarms are not critical, they are important because they could indicate danger with the patient. They are reduced and silenced as much as possible. The ICU team is sorry for whatever disturbance they may cause, especially during those night hours.

Nurse's Note

- Alert the nurse if the monitor is sounding an alarm.

Figure 3.1   The Monitor

The monitor shows the patient's vital signs and other important information. Depending on the illness, patients may have more or less information displayed on their monitor.

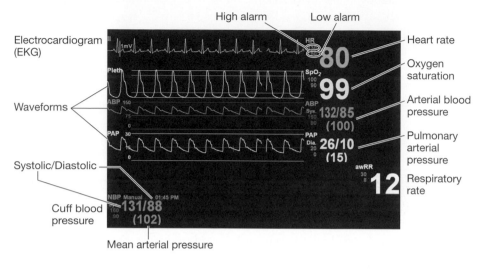

Intravenous Access

Every ICU patient needs <u>intravenous (IV) access</u>. It is used to draw blood and give most medications and fluids. Also called a peripheral IV (PIV), it is a plastic tube that usually is inserted into a vein of the hand, forearm, or inside of the elbow. The nurse inserts the IV and flushes it with saline fluid regularly to make sure it is working. An IV lasts about a week until it has to be taken out. The dressing fully covers where the IV enters the skin and is kept clean and dry.

Typically, an ICU patient needs at least two IVs. This is to prevent needing IV access in an emergency. It is safer to have two IVs in case one stops working or more than one is needed.

Nurse's Note

- If you know which areas are easier or harder for an IV to be placed, tell the nurse before it is inserted.
- You may be more comfortable if the IV is inserted in your nondominant forearm. However, it may have to be placed wherever it is possible.
- Alert the nurse if the IV area is swollen, red, hurts, or leaks fluid.
- Even if an IV does not draw blood, it may still work fine for giving fluids and medication. If this happens, the medical team may have to draw blood with a needle for labs. Please see Lab Tests for more information (page 61).
- If it is hard to insert IVs in you, it may be worth discussing a midline or a peripherally inserted central catheter (PICC) with the medical team (page 38). These offer more reliable IV access, so you will be poked less.

Figure 3.2 Peripheral IV Examples

Pictured are some of the many types of Peripheral IVs. They are usually placed between the hand and the bicep. Typically, an ICU patient needs two, and it is flushed with saline periodically to make sure it works.

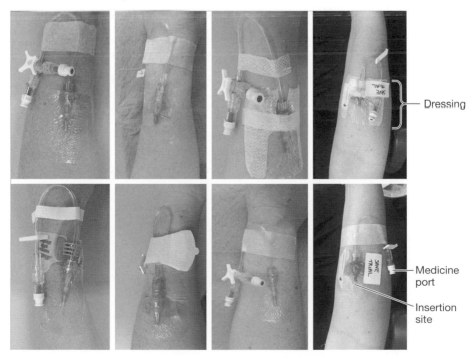

Dressing

Medicine port

Insertion site

Medication Pumps

Medication pumps, also known as infusion pumps, are programmed to deliver the right amount of medication in a set amount of time. The tubing is connected to an IV tube that enters the vein of the patient. This is how the medication flows into the bloodstream. Unfortunately, they are another source of tubing and alarms.

Nurse's Note

- Never push any buttons on this, or any, machine.
- Sometimes, IVs are inserted into the patient's wrist or inside the elbow. These may be annoying because, if you imagine your veins like a hose with water running through it, every time you bend that spot, the hose will kink. The pumps are sensitive and alarm when this happens. If this is a problem, you can remind your family member to straighten their arm or wrist when the alarm is heard. You can also ask the nurse to use another IV that is less problematic.

Figure 3.3 Medication Pumps

These pumps give the patient medication through the IV. Please let the nurse know if it is alarming, and do not touch any of the buttons.

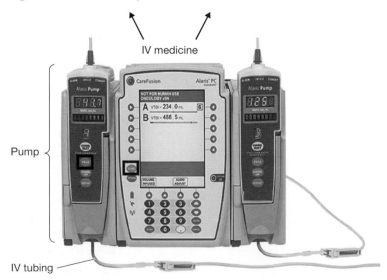

Computers and Electronic Medical Records

Computers and the electronic medical records (EMR) are critical to the job of all the ICU team members. The EMR can tell the medications that have to be given, the history of the patient, the laboratory results, and much more. It is important because it makes patient care better and helps to prevent mistakes. However, the downside is that everything has to be documented multiple times a day into the EMR. Therefore, please forgive the medical team while they are looking at the screen.

Prefer Another Language

All hospitals are required by law to provide translation and interpretation for all patients. If English is not the preferred language, please request a translator. It makes the hospital experience safer and easier for the patient, family, and medical team.

Visiting the Patient

Each hospital has their own rules for visiting a patient. Typically, there is a limit to how many people can visit, when visiting hours are, and how long visitors can stay at the bedside. Additionally, there may be a minimum age limit. Anyone who is feeling ill should not visit. These rules are important to help all the patients rest and recover. Please ask the nurse what the visitation rules are, so the expectations are made clear as early as possible. Even if the family has experience with the hospital, these guidelines change frequently. The ICU team thanks the family for working to help keep the patients safe.

Nurse's Note

- Please do not visit if you are sick. This puts patients in danger of catching another illness.
- Many ICUs have rules about family staying in the patient's room and not roaming around the unit. This is to protect the privacy of all patients and to keep the halls clear in case of emergency situations. Please do not be surprised or offended if you are asked to either step back in the room or go into the waiting area until you are ready to return to the room.
- Exceptions to the visitation policy are made on a case-by-case basis. Most exceptions are only made for end-of-life scenarios. You can ask the nurse to see if an exception can be made.

Preventing Infection

Unfortunately, the equipment necessary for treatment in the ICU increases the risk of infection. Where the lines, tubes, and drains enter the body are where germs can grow. If the germs travel into the body, an infection can occur. Because this can harm the patient, preventing infection is built into everything the ICU staff does.

Each ICU has rules for preventing germs from growing, such as performing procedures sterilely, cleaning urinary catheters, and regularly changing dressings (protective covering over an IV or drain). Additionally, the healthcare team is always assessing for signs of an infection. This may be suspected when there is redness or pain where an IV or tube enters the body, when a fever occurs, or when more white blood cells are measured in the blood.

Because anyone can spread germs, each person plays an important role in preventing infection. To help with this, a set of rules are in place that everyone has to follow. These rules are called standard precautions (SP) or universal precautions. A central part of SP is clean hands, which is the best way to prevent infection. Everyone—family as well as staff—has to use soap and water or the hand sanitizer, at minimum:

- When entering the patient's room
- When leaving the patient's room
- After all contact with the patient
- After handling equipment

Additionally, any time hands are dirty, like after covering a cough or sneeze, hand cleaning should occur. Gloves are usually only worn by the staff, but the nurse can advise family at the bedside. These protections work and are the minimum requirements everyone has to follow.

When a patient has an infection that can be given to the staff, other patients, or visitors, extra steps are taken to protect those in the room. Extra protective gear, known as personal protective equipment (PPE), may be required. The PPE needed depends on what the infection is and how it can spread. This can include a gown, gloves, eye protection, and a mask.

Importantly, SP are needed in all cases. If there are any questions, the nurse can explain what is necessary. Although a hassle, the only thing families want to bring home from the hospital is the patient.

Nurse's Note

- Usually, a sign is hanging outside of the patient's room indicating what type of PPE is required. You can always ask the nurse if you are unsure of what to wear or for how long.
- PPE needs to be worn the entire time you are in the patient's room.
- To keep yourself and the patient safe, make sure that everyone is following the precautions.

Figure 3.4 Infection Prevention Sign

A sign like this will be outside the patient's room if personal protective equipment is needed to enter.

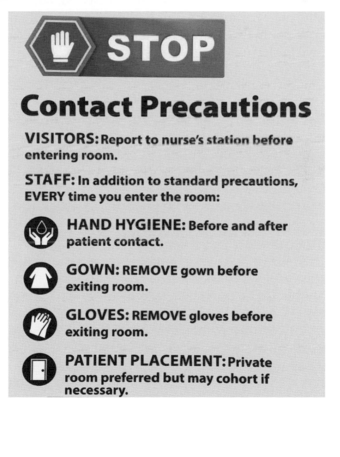

Transfer Out of the ICU

When patients do not need lifesaving medical care, they will be transferred to another unit. This floor can be called a progressive care unit, stepdown, telemetry, acute care, the floor, or have another name. This decision is made by the providers.

The ICU provider and nurse update the provider and nurse of the new unit so they are familiar with the patient, and therapists continue to provide care. Some patients worry because they will not have the level of supervision that comes with being in the ICU. This is a common concern but there are reasons to not be upset. First, the medical team would not transfer someone who is too sick to leave the ICU. Second, the staff on those floors know how to best care for patients transferred from the ICU. Third, patients tend to like them better because the staff bothers them less often. This is one step closer to leaving the hospital, and usually the patients enjoy being able to sleep throughout most of the night.

4

Common Procedures

Consent, Capacity, and Important Questions

Many procedures occur in the intensive care unit (ICU). Some of these procedures require the patient to confirm that they want the treatment. If the patient cannot make a choice, their durable power of attorney (DPOA) assumes this role. The next section explains these scenarios and presents questions to ask in order to make the best decision. Information about a DPOA is covered in Goals of Care (page 137).

Informed Consent—Explaining All the Options

When a provider believes a procedure or treatment is needed to help a patient, they are required to obtain the patient's <u>informed consent</u>. This is when the provider discusses the benefits and burdens of all the possible treatments in a way that is personalized, culturally sensitive, and in the patient's preferred language. What may happen if no treatment is given is also covered. The patient then chooses which option, if any, they prefer.

The decision should be made voluntarily, and the patient should have capacity to do so, which is discussed in the following

Capacity section. Once a decision is made, the patient is asked to sign a form saying the informed consent was appropriately obtained.

Nurse's Note

■ It is OK to ask for the medical team's recommendation and to include trusted family in this conversation.

■ It is OK to refuse the medical team's recommendation. They may ask how you came to that decision so they can understand your reasoning.

■ Not all treatments and procedures require informed consent. But, you can still ask the questions given below for your own informed consent.

■ An additional informed consent has to be signed again for a treatment agreed to in a previous admission. This is to make sure you are presently informed, and your choice of treatment has not changed.

■ When making decisions for the patient (if you are their durable power of attorney), the therapies chosen for the patient should align with their goals of care. Therefore, the patient's desires should direct the consent. Please see Goals of Care (page 137) for more on this.

■ In an emergency, consent from the patient or family may not be obtained if two providers agree that the procedure is appropriate and necessary for life. If the patient has preferences for their medical care in an emergency, you should let the medical team know. Please see Goals of Care (page 135) for more on this.

Questions to Ask for Informed Consent
■ Why is medical help needed?
■ What are the options for treatment that align with the patient's goals of care?
  ● Procedure vs medicine vs wait and see vs combination?
■ For each option:
  ● What is the most likely outcome for similar patients?
  ● What is the best-case scenario and how common is it?
  ● What is the worst-case scenario and how common is it?
  ● How is the patient recovery and family experience in the short- and long-term?
  ● How often do the risks happen during and after?
■ What do both the patient and family need to think about moving forward?
■ When does a decision need to be made?

Capacity—Can the Patient Make Their Own Decisions?

ICU patients can be confused, sedated, or unable to communicate. This is a problem when decisions about treatment are needed.

In these cases, patients may not be able to choose the medical care that supports their goals. To ensure the right decisions are being made, the ICU staff has to determine if each patient has the ability to make an informed decision.

What indicates this is called <u>capacity</u>, which is sometimes called competency. This a combination of abilities. Patients with capacity are able to communicate what the details of their illness are, what can occur going forward with and without treatment, and why the medical team is recommending one option over another.

When a decision needs to be made, capacitated patients are able to understand the details, reason through each option, and make a logical choice based on their current illness.

Every effort should be made to improve the patient's capacity. For instance, try to time the discussion for when the patient is usually most active and alert. Before the talk, a cup of coffee and prepping the patient for what is to come can prime their reasoning abilities. Importantly, suggesting what the "correct" decision is should be avoided. The better option is to review the choices to think through so the patient's readiness is improved.

Correcting dehydration, fever, confusion, and delirium are all helpful in boosting capacity as well. Additionally, the family, patient, and medical team should work together to avoid medications that can cause confusion. Mental illnesses, such as anxiety and depression, may also affect capacity. The medical team can involve specialists, such as the ethics committee or a psychologist, for complicated scenarios. Furthermore, just because a patient lacks capacity now does not mean they will lack it later. It is necessary to assess this at each point in the decision-making process.

Additionally, if a patient does not possess capacity at one point in time about a single question, it does not mean they lack capacity about everything at that point. A complex issue can be revisited later, but simpler decisions may be manageable now, such as wanting pain medicine.

It is important to understand that patients with capacity have the right to choose what some may view as the "wrong" option. However, this decision should follow the patient's values and beliefs about what is important to them. The communication of these decisions and the discussion between the patient, family, and provider are the critical pieces.

When a patient lacks capacity, the DPOA is empowered to make the decision. Who this is and considerations at this point are covered in Goals of Care (page 137).

Nurse's Note

- Family can help prevent confusion by reminding the patient of the day, time, where they are, what is going on, etc, but they should not try to influence the patient. Patients should be free to make their own decision and include their family if they choose.
- Ask the nurse or providers to schedule the informed consent and capacity discussion at the patient's optimal time. Unfortunately, this may not be an option in emergencies.
- Before an informed consent or capacity conversation, create a good decision-making environment. Turn off the TV, turn on the lights, drink coffee/tea, review possibilities for the decision, minimize pain, use the restroom, inform all necessary participants of the time for the meeting, ask to discuss after a rest if tired, wear hearing aids and glasses if necessary, and avoid the talk during mealtimes.
- If the patient still has capacity and has chosen you as the DPOA, ask which therapies they would want if they cannot make their own decisions. Please see Goals of Care (page 135) for more on this.

The Procedures

The following are procedures the patient may experience. After each procedure is described, three bullet points follow. The first bullet point is who carries out the procedure. The second is the reasons for the procedure. The third features tips for the family and patient. It should be noted that the type of provider that performs the procedure and equipment used may differ depending on the hospital. Many procedures occur with sterile precautions (see Sterile Procedures, page 46). Please see NavigatingTheICU.com for more information about these procedures.

Arterial Line

An arterial line (A-line) is used to measure blood pressure continuously and to allow easy and reliable access to blood for lab tests. It is a small catheter (tube), like an IV, inserted into the wrist or groin under sterile precautions.

In critically ill patients, blood pressure can drop rapidly. In these situations, a specific amount of a medication, known as a vasopressor, needs to be given to increase blood pressure. Alternatively, some situations require keeping blood pressure in a certain range so that no organ damage occurs. The blood pressure cuff can take too long in an emergency, so the instant blood pressure reading of the arterial line is preferred. Additionally, it allows access to blood so the patient does not have to be stuck with a needle for each sample.

Because the arterial blood flow comes straight from the heart, it is highly pressurized. If the line is pulled out unnoticed, the patient can bleed to death. Thus, care needs to be taken when moving to prevent accidental removal. Alarms will notify the nurse if this happens, but it is best to be careful. Furthermore, the nurse needs to hold pressure on the site for about 10 minutes when removing the arterial line, which can be uncomfortable. Distractions can help the time pass, like turning on the TV, listening to music, practicing breathing exercises, etc.

- Who Performs the Procedure
  - A provider or respiratory therapist.
- Its Purpose
  - Real-time blood pressure measurement and blood draws.
- Family Participation
  - Will need to wait outside to ensure the procedure is sterile.
  - Be careful when moving to avoid pulling out the line.
  - Let the nurse know if the dressing is falling off to help prevent infection.
  - Keep an eye out for bleeding, redness, or discharge where it enters the body.
  - Consent needed.

Figure 4.1   Arterial Line

The arterial line allows for continuous blood pressure monitoring and easy blood draws. Usually, it is placed in the radial artery, below the palm of the hand. It is connected to tubing and a saline bag that is hung close to the patient.

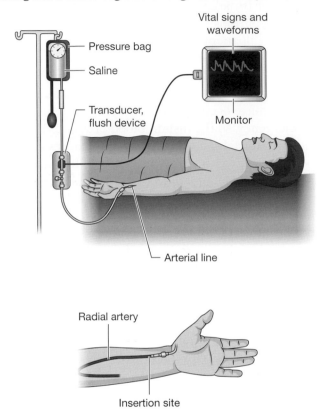

Blood Transfusion

A blood transfusion, where blood from a donor is given to the patient through an IV, is common in the ICU. The ability to do this safely is essential in any ICU, and improvements in matching the patient's blood with the donor's have nearly eliminated all danger. Furthermore, because donated blood is thoroughly screened for any viruses or bacteria, infection from a blood transfusion is very rare.

Each ICU has its own way for giving blood. However, they all begin by taking the patient's blood and sending it to the lab to determine their blood type. The matching blood is then sent to the nurse for administration.

When blood is donated, the different parts that make up blood are separated. The different parts are called blood products. The types of blood products are packed red blood cells (PRBCs), fresh frozen plasma (FFP), platelets, and cryoprecipitate. Each of these four blood products is useful for different scenarios.

- PRBCs provide the ability to carry oxygen to tissues and increase blood pressure by adding more fluid in the veins.
  - Given when a patient does not have enough red blood cells due to bleeding, surgery, or anemia.
  - Given when a patient has low blood pressure because there is not enough blood, such as when bleeding.
  - This is the most commonly transfused blood product.
- FFP provides clotting abilities that help to stop bleeding. It increases blood pressure by adding more fluid in the veins. If needed to fight an infection, antibodies (the body's defenders) are included.
  - Given when a patient has low blood pressure because there is not enough blood, such as when bleeding.
  - Given when a patient's blood does not have enough of the ingredients to clot in order to stop or prevent bleeding.
  - Given to patients with low clotting abilities before a procedure to help them stop a bleed if it occurs.
  - Given to help fight infections.
- Platelets provide clotting abilities that help to stop bleeding.
  - Given to patients with low platelet levels to help their blood clot in order to stop or prevent bleeding.
  - Given to patients with low platelet levels before a procedure to help them stop a bleed if it occurs.
- Cryoprecipitate provides clotting abilities that help to stop bleeding.
  - Given when a patient's blood does not have enough of the ingredients to clot in order to stop or prevent bleeding.

The nurse monitors the patient closely for any signs or symptoms of bad reactions to the donor's blood. Although generally very safe, it is important to be aware of these signs because they can indicate danger. A mild reaction, with the patient getting itchy and developing a fever, is possible. Medications reduce these symptoms so the patient is able to receive the needed blood products. Signs of serious reactions include trouble breathing, back pain, swelling, or anxiety. If any of these symptoms occur either during or after the transfusion, the ICU staff needs to be alerted IMMEDIATELY. The transfusion is stopped, the symptoms are treated, and an even closer watch is kept on the patient. The blood product is sent to the lab to see why it caused the reaction, and the patient receives another transfusion.

- ■ Who Performs the Procedure
  - ● A nurse.
- ■ Its Purpose
  - ● Supplement the necessary parts of blood, usually to support blood pressure, stop or prevent bleeding, or increase the blood's ability to carry oxygen to tissues.
- ■ Family Participation
  - ● IMMEDIATELY report anything new or different to the nurse, including flushing (turning red), feeling hot, itchiness, trouble breathing, pain, anxiety, or swelling.
  - ● If you have a history of transfusion reactions, please let the staff know so they can give medication to avoid uncomfortable reactions.
  - ● Consent needed.

Bronchoscopy

If a patient is having trouble breathing, coughing up fluid, or needs a sample taken (biopsy), a bronchoscopy may be considered. This procedure allows the caregivers to see inside the lungs and suck out fluid or mucus to help the patient breathe. That fluid can be examined to see if an infection is present. Additionally, if there is a blockage, the object can be removed.

Completed under moderate sedation (see page 57), the patient is made comfortable with medication to reduce pain, anxiety, and memory formation during the procedure. A small tube with a camera and light is inserted through the mouth and into the lungs. The provider assesses the airways, removes fluids, etc, while the nurse or anesthesia provider takes care of the patient by administering the medications and monitoring vital signs. This usually lasts around 15 minutes, and the patient returns to preprocedure form about an hour after it is completed.

- ■ Who Performs the Procedure
  - ● A provider and nurse.
- ■ Its Purpose
  - ● To view the lungs, sample fluid or tissue, and remove blockages.
- ■ Family Participation
  - ● Family may prefer to wait outside.
  - ● Consent needed.

Figure 4.2 Bronchoscopy

A bronchoscope can see inside the patient's lungs and remove any blockages with an instrument. During the procedure, the patient is sedated so minimal discomfort is felt.

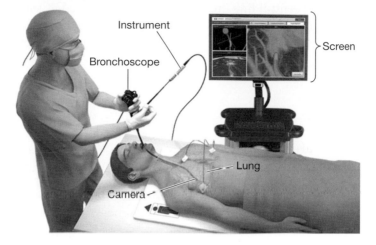

Central Line

Peripheral intravenous tubes (IVs) are inserted into small veins and last about a week. Although these IVs work for many situations, some medications can damage those small veins. Also, some patients may benefit from another type of IV that lasts longer.

A dependable way to give medications and draw blood is the central line, which is placed deep in a large vein of the neck, chest, or groin. Also called a central venous catheter, this tube is inserted by a provider at the bedside. The area is first numbed with medication, and the vein is visualized with an ultrasound machine. To prevent infection, the entire process is sterile. The correct placement in the neck or chest is confirmed with an X-ray before use. This is because the end of the line will be just outside the entrance of the heart. If touching the walls of the heart, the catheter can cause irregular heartbeats, known as arrhythmias.

Another use for a central line is to provide nutrition to patients who cannot tolerate food through their stomach or intestines. For these patients, nutrition can be directly injected into their bloodstream through this IV, termed total parenteral nutrition (TPN). Additionally, if dialysis is needed, it will usually take place through a similar central line.

Not all patients in the ICU need central lines, and not all central lines are needed for a long time. Importantly, the ICU team takes out the line when it is no longer needed to prevent infection. Infections from these lines can be devastating. They go into a big vein near the heart. If the line becomes infected, these germs can get washed into the bloodstream where they grow. This is called a central line–associated bloodstream infection (CLABSI) and can be deadly. To avoid infection, the central line dressing should be changed at least every 7 days, when dirty, or when the insertion site (where the line enters the body) is uncovered. These dressing changes are done sterilely.

- ■ Who Performs the Procedure
  - ● A provider.
- ■ Its Purpose
  - ● Reliable access for all medications, TPN, dialysis, and blood draws.
- ■ Family Participation
  - ● Will need to wait outside to ensure the procedure is sterile.
  - ● Let the nurse know if the dressing is falling off, wet, or dirty. It may need to be replaced to prevent infection.
  - ● Tell the nurse if there is bleeding, soreness, redness, or discharge around the insertion site.
  - ● Consent needed.

Figure 4.3   Central Line

The central line catheter is inserted into a large vein in the neck, chest, or groin. If inserted into the neck (as pictured) or chest, the catheter ends just outside the heart.

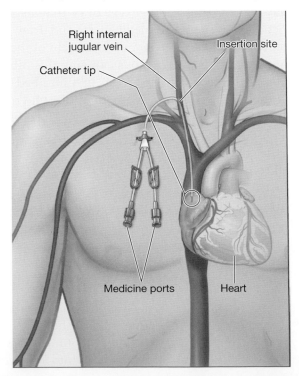

Figure 4.4 Central Line Dressing

The central line dressing should be clean and cover the insertion site. Many hospitals place an antibiotic patch or film around the insertion site to prevent infections.

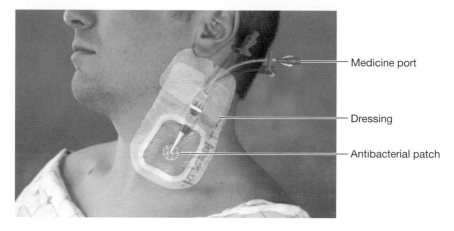

Medicine port

Dressing

Antibacterial patch

Chest Tube

If air or fluid builds up around the lungs, the patient cannot take full breaths. To help the patient breathe, a chest tube, or thoracostomy tube, may be required to drain what is compressing the lungs. This tube drains the air or fluid into a container, called an atrium. The lungs can then fully open.

Pain medicine is given before inserting the chest tube, which occurs at the bedside. If the patient is undergoing a heart or lung surgery, a few chest tubes may be inserted in the operating room (OR). This thin plastic tube is inserted between the ribs and into the space surrounding the lungs, called the pleural space. It is stitched into place and connected to the drainage system. Suction is sometimes used to help drain the air or fluid. The system is monitored for any drainage or air leaks. The nurse cleans the site where it enters the skin and replaces the dressing regularly to prevent infection. Although it may be painful, the patient should try to breathe deeply. Pain around the insertion site and in the shoulder are common, and lidocaine patches, acetaminophen, and nonsteroidal anti-inflammatory drugs (NSAIDs) may provide relief. When the lungs have expanded and the drainage is minimal, the chest tube is removed at the bedside. This occurs quickly and can briefly cause discomfort.

- Who Performs the Procedure
  - A provider.
- Its Purpose
  - Remove air and fluid from around the lungs.

■ Family Participation
  ● Will need to wait outside to ensure the insertion is sterile.
  ● Report pain, trouble breathing, or swelling around the neck and face immediately.
  ● Be mindful of the collection device, which is often placed on the floor around the bed.
  ● Consent needed.

Figure 4.5   Chest Tube and Atrium

A chest tube is inserted into the space around the lung to drain fluid or air. The chest tube connects to an atrium, where the collected fluid can be measured. The atrium is usually next to the bed and connected to suction tubing.

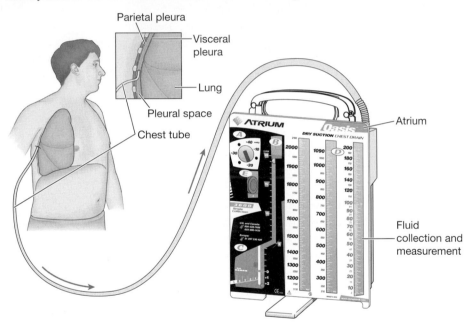

Esophagogastroduodenoscopy

An esophagogastroduodenoscopy, typically referred to as an EGD or upper endoscopy, is a procedure that is used to visualize the throat (esophagus), stomach (gastric), and small intestine (duodenum). Usually, this test is needed if there are any signs of bleeding, such as blood in the vomit or stool. Tissue samples can also be taken to see if this area is healthy.

The patient may not be allowed to eat for some time before the EGD. Completed under moderate sedation (see page 57), the patient is made comfortable with medication to reduce pain, anxiety, and memory formation during the procedure. A nurse or anesthesia provider administers the medication and closely tracks the patient's vital signs. A provider then passes an endoscope, a thin tube with a camera, through the mouth, down the throat, and into the stomach. The images from the endoscope can be seen on a screen next to the provider. To stop any bleeding, the provider can insert tools through the endoscope to pinch the area closed, burn the leaking blood vessel, or inject medication around the site. Another EGD may be required later to make sure the bleeding has stopped.

The procedure lasts about 30 minutes, and the patient should return to preprocedure form after about an hour. A sore throat and sleepiness are common but should not last more than a couple hours. After the procedure, patients may only be allowed to eat clear liquids (jello, juice, broth, etc) to protect the EGD area and prevent nausea and vomiting.

- Who Performs the Procedure
  - A provider.
- Its Purpose
  - Examine the throat, stomach, and small intestine, stop bleeding, and take tissue samples.
- Family Participation
  - Family may prefer to wait outside.
  - Monitor for signs of bleeding, such as blood in vomit or dark, tarry stool.
  - Consent needed.

Figure 4.6   Esophagogastroduodenoscopy (EGD) or Upper Endoscopy

An EGD typically is used to look for and stop any bleeding in the throat, stomach, and small intestine. During the procedure, the patient is sedated so minimal discomfort is felt.

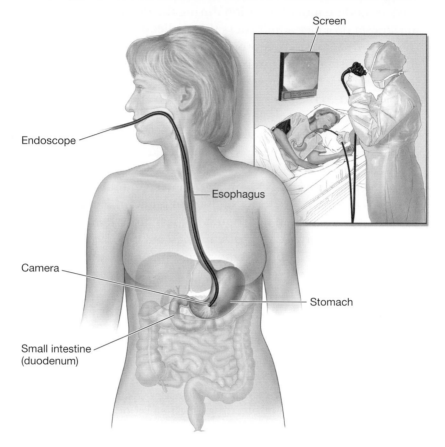

Feeding Tube for the Short Term—Nasogastric, Orogastric, and Nasoduodenal Tubes

If a patient is unable to swallow safely, requires more calories or hydration, has a breathing tube, or needs stomach contents to be removed, a feeding tube is discussed. This tube is inserted either through the nose (nasogastric, or NG) or mouth (orogastric, or OG) and ends in the stomach. The OG is preferred for patients with a breathing tube. The NG is preferred in patients without a breathing tube because it does not interfere with speaking.

Inserting an NG tube can be uncomfortable, but should not be painful. After sitting the patient up in bed, lubrication is applied to the tube, and it is guided through the back of the nose where it reaches the throat. The patient then is asked to swallow while the nurse glides the tube into the stomach. The nurse must confirm the tube's correct placement by injecting air while listening to the stomach for a "whoosh" sound, drawing back stomach contents with a syringe, or taking an X-ray. This tube is taped to the nose, and numbers on it tell the staff how deep it goes.

A nasoduodenal (ND) tube enters through the nose, passes through the stomach, and ends in the small intestine. Ending past the stomach prevents patients from breathing in stomach contents that have traveled up the throat. This is known as aspiration and can cause a lung infection. The ND is also smaller and less likely to cause pressure injuries than the OG or NG, so it can be tolerated for longer. It is inserted similarly to the NG, and the correct ND placement is confirmed with an X-ray. Numbers on it tell the staff how deep it goes, and it is taped to the nose. Because it ends past the stomach, the ND cannot be used to remove stomach contents. If the patient continues to pull it out, the ND can be secured, or bridled, to the nose with a string.

A liquid, referred to as tube feeds, is pumped through the OG, NG, or ND and provides the patient's nutrition.

- Who Performs the Procedure
  - A nurse.
- Its Purpose
  - Feeding, hydration, medication administration, or removal of stomach contents.
- Family Participation
  - Provide support during the tube's placement.
  - Monitor for signs of redness or skin breakdown.
  - Encourage the patient to not touch or pull on this tube.

Figure 4.7 Feeding Tube Options

The different types of short- and long-term feeding tubes are shown. Depending on the patient, they may be used for nutrition, hydration, medication administration, or removing stomach contents.

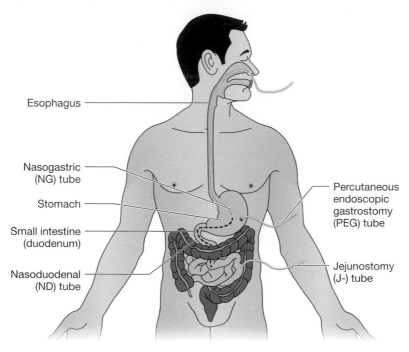

Feeding Tube for the Long Term—Percutaneous Endoscopic Gastrostomy and Gastrostomy/Jejunostomy Tubes

More permanent access to the stomach is necessary if long-term tube feeding is required. Patients are considered for this procedure if they have not recovered the ability to swallow or they remain on a ventilator for over 2 weeks. If used for an extended period, the OG, NG, and ND might cause pressure injuries and increase the risk of stomach contents traveling into the lungs. They can also be annoying, which causes some patients to remove them.

A percutaneous endoscopic gastrostomy (PEG, "peg") tube provides a secured entrance directly into the stomach that allows for long-term tube feedings. It is inserted under sedation, usually in the OR, so the patient is comfortable. A camera (endoscope) is passed through the mouth into the stomach, and a light is shone toward the front of the stomach. Where the light can be seen shining through the abdominal skin is where a small hole is made to allow the tube access into the stomach. It can be used for medicine four hours after the insertion, and tube feedings can begin after about a day.

Gastrostomy/jejunostomy (G/J) tubes have two ports, one that accesses the stomach (gastro/G) and one that accesses the small intestine (jejuno/J). Access to the small intestine—the J side—decreases the risk of aspiration. Typically, tube feed nutrition goes through the J side, while medications go into the stomach through the G side.

- Who Performs the Procedure
  - A provider.
- Its Purpose
  - Long-term tube feeding, hydration, medication administration, or removal of stomach contents.
- Family Participation
  - Monitor for signs of leaking or skin redness.
  - Learn from the nurse how to manage care because this device may be used after leaving the hospital.
  - Consent needed.

Please see Figure 4.7 for the feeding tube options.

Figure 4.8 Percutaneous Endoscopic Gastrostomy (PEG) Tube Insertion

A PEG tube enables a long-term way to give nutrition to a patient. It is usually placed in the OR with the help of an endoscope.

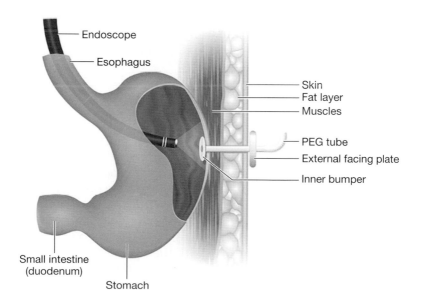

Peripherally Inserted Central Catheter

Some patients require a long-term IV for antibiotics, chemotherapy, IV nutrition (total parenteral nutrition), or frequent blood draws. In these cases, a peripherally inserted central catheter (PICC, "pick") is recommended.

This central line typically is inserted in a vein near the patient's bicep and guided to just outside the entrance of the heart. A provider or specialized nurse does this at the bedside.

Nurse's Note

■ Because a central line infection can be dangerous, a safer option may be a midline catheter. A midline is shorter than a PICC, but longer than a regular peripheral IV. This makes for a safe way to have consistent IV access, while lowering the risk of infection. Therefore, a midline may be a good option to discuss if it is hard to place an IV in the patient or if the patient needs a longer-term IV. However, it is not suitable for all medications.

This is a sterile procedure, and the medical team confirms the correct catheter location before use. It can remain in place for months, so long as there are no complications. The nurse or provider gives patients and their families guidance about proper care at the time of insertion. Two important rules are to not get the area wet and to monitor the area for signs of infection.

- Who Performs the Procedure
  - A provider or specialized nurse.
- Its Purpose
  - Reliable, long-term access for all medications, TPN, and blood draws.
- Family Participation
  - Will need to wait outside to ensure the procedure is sterile.
  - Let the nurse know if the dressing is falling off, wet, or dirty. It may need to be replaced to prevent infection.
  - Tell the nurse if you see bleeding, soreness, redness, or discharge around the insertion site.
  - Report swelling of the arm with the PICC.
  - Notify the nurse if there is a change in the length of catheter coming from the insertion site.
  - Consent needed.

Figure 4.9 Peripherally Inserted Central Catheter (PICC) and Midline Catheter

A long-term central line, the PICC allows for administration of IV medications, TPN, and enables blood draws. The midline catheter may be a safer option, but may not be appropriate for all patients.

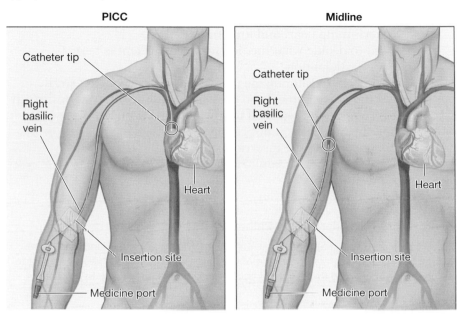

Pulmonary Artery Catheter

A pulmonary artery catheter (Swan-Ganz catheter, PA catheter) may be recommended for patients with heart or lung issues. This not only provides the abilities of a central line, but also allows the ICU staff to use a pressure sensor to measure how well the heart and lungs are functioning.

Usually inserted into a vein in the neck, the catheter is advanced further than a typical central line. It has a balloon on the tip that can be inflated. When the catheter is directly outside the heart, the balloon is inflated. It passes through the opening of the heart, the right atrium, the right ventricle and into the pulmonary artery. If touching the walls of the heart, the catheter can cause irregular heartbeats, known as arrhythmias. Throughout the placement, the catheter is visualized by x-rays or ultrasound to confirm its location. The medical team also can tell where the tip of the catheter is by the pressure changes sensed as it passes through the different chambers of the heart. These numbers tell the ICU staff about the functioning of the heart and lungs. Additionally, these readings help determine which treatments will best help the patient.

- Who Performs the Procedure
  - A provider.
- Its Purpose
  - Reliable access for all medications, TPN, and blood draws.
  - Determining heart and lung functioning.
  - Used to decide what medication or treatment is best.
- Family Participation
  - Will need to wait outside to ensure the procedure is sterile.
  - Let the nurse know if the dressing is falling off, wet, or dirty. It may need to be replaced to prevent infection.
  - Tell the nurse if you notice bleeding, soreness, redness, or discharge around the insertion site.
  - Report any new irregular heartbeats to the nurse.
  - Consent needed.

Figure 4.10   Pulmonary Artery Catheter

The pulmonary artery catheter tells how well the heart and lungs are functioning. The catheter is guided through the right side of the heart and into a blood vessel leading to the lungs. It is connected to tubing and a saline bag that is hung close to the patient.

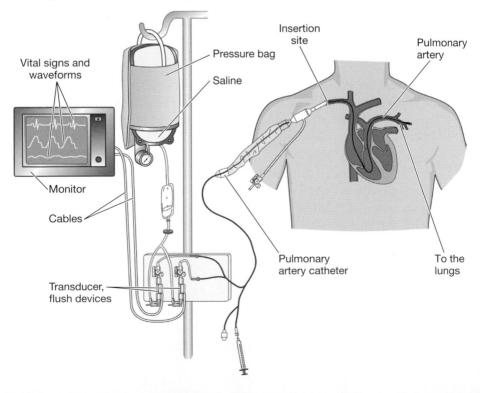

Swallow Test

When patients have a breathing tube removed, suffer a stroke, or are not very alert, they have an increased risk of aspiration. Aspirating (getting food or liquids in the lungs) can result in a dangerous lung infection. To prevent this, a swallow test is needed.

Typically, the nurse sits a fully awake patient up and gives them a cup of water to drink. To pass the swallow test, a patient must be able to drink without choking or coughing and be able to speak normally after. If the patient coughs, chokes, or has trouble speaking, they cannot have anything to eat or drink for now. This is known as being NPO (see page 120).

The next step is a formal evaluation by the speech-language pathologist (SLP). They will examine all things related to the patient's ability to safely eat and drink. The SLP tests the patient's ability to swallow different consistencies of food and liquid and suggests strategies for how to safely eat and drink. For example, the patient may be able to handle honey-consistency liquids and softer foods only if fully awake and sitting up in bed. The SLP's swallowing assessment can be repeated every day or so. If there is too much risk of aspiration or the patient cannot consume enough calories needed for recovery, tube feeding may be considered.

- Who Performs the Procedure
  - A nurse. If further help is needed, a speech-language pathologist.
- Its Purpose
  - To see if a patient can safely swallow and if help is needed for eating or drinking.
- Family Participation
  - Family is most important after the test because the safety instructions for eating and drinking are needed for each and every bite and sip.
  - Once patients have passed a swallow test, only allow them food and water if they are sitting upright and are fully awake!
  - Be sure to follow the SLP's instructions for <u>how</u> to eat and drink.
  - If the patient has a new cough or is having trouble breathing after eating or drinking, let the nurse know.
  - This is different than a barium swallow test, also known as a swallow study, which may be recommended if the patient continues to have difficulty swallowing.

Tracheostomy

A tracheostomy, or trach, is a hole created in the front of the neck for access to the windpipe, or trachea. This procedure is done for three reasons, and all of them aim to improve breathing.

The first reason a trach is needed is to bypass an obstruction, such as airway swelling. The second reason is to help remove saliva and mucous (secretions). This is common in patients who have a weak cough, such as those who are paralyzed. These patients cannot cough up secretions as they build up in their trachea. This makes it harder to breathe and blocks air from entering their lungs. Inhaling those secretions also increases the risk of a lung infection. The trach creates the ability to remove those secretions.

The third and most common reason for a trach is a prolonged need for the breathing machine (ventilator). After a patient has spent about 2 weeks on the ventilator, a tracheostomy is discussed (this can only happen if the amount of oxygen and breathing support needed are low enough). The breathing tube can be uncomfortable and increase the risk of pressure injuries. A trach safely allows for more comfortable breathing assistance from the ventilator than through the breathing tube. As a result, the medical team can use less medicine to relax the patient, and it may reduce the amount of breathing assistance the patient needs. Hopefully, this will make the patient more awake and able to interact.

The patient and family should discuss the changes a tracheostomy brings with the nurse, respiratory therapist, provider, and social worker. Although plenty of people care for tracheostomies on their own, it requires frequent maintenance. Importantly, a trach can be removed if the ability to safely breathe is regained.

This procedure is performed either at the bedside under moderate sedation or in the OR under general sedation. A surgical hole, known as a stoma, is created in the trachea on the front of the neck. An outer tube called a cannula is inserted and secured with stitches to keep the stoma open. An inner cannula, which can be changed and cleaned, is inserted within the outer cannula. Usually, it takes about a week for the stoma to heal and for the stitches to be removed.

The nurse and respiratory therapist care for the trach site. These tasks include cleaning, changing the dressing around the trach, suctioning secretions, and replacing the inner cannula. Some of these tasks occur when they are needed, like suctioning, and others are scheduled.

Nurse's Note

▪ Try to get a feel for the maintenance of the trach from the nurse or RT because care after the hospital is similar.

▪ It is normal for a new trach to ooze blood as it heals. If it is affecting the ability to breathe, then let the nurse know.

Communication is difficult after the insertion of a trach because the patient cannot speak. Different strategies have to be practiced for communicating until the patient can use their voice with a speaking valve. Some of these include writing, texting on a phone, reading lips, or using a communication board. The nurse and speech-language pathologist can provide strategies during this time to help make this experience less frustrating.

The patient can learn how to speak with a speaking valve once full-time breathing assistance is not needed. This one-way valve allows air in, and the patient forces the air over the vocal cords and out of the mouth to speak. The speaking and swallowing muscles, made weak from lack of use, need to be strengthened with help from a speech-language pathologist. Until the ability to safely eat is regained, nutrition is given through a feeding tube or IV. The ICU team can provide much more information on this topic.

- Who Performs the Procedure
  - A provider.
- Its Purpose
  - Bypass blockage, remove secretions, and provide long-term breathing support.
- Family Participation
  - Will need to wait outside to ensure the procedure is sterile (if occurring at the bedside).
  - Nurses, respiratory therapists, and speech-language pathologists are great resources.
  - Learn the maintenance of a trach.
  - Talk to a social worker about support groups for people with trachs.
  - Consent needed.

Figure 4.11 Tracheostomy

A tracheostomy helps the patient breathe. It can also reduce the need for sedation medication, which will allow the patient to be more active.

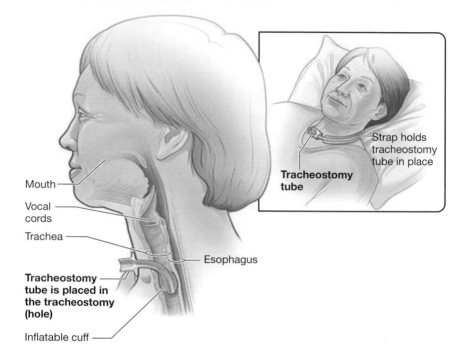

Mouth

Vocal cords

Trachea

Esophagus

Tracheostomy tube is placed in the tracheostomy (hole)

Inflatable cuff

Strap holds tracheostomy tube in place

Tracheostomy tube

Urinary Catheter

There are many reasons to use a urinary catheter, or Foley, to drain the bladder. The catheter temporarily relieves urinary retention, bypasses the blockage of an enlarged prostate, and prevents the development and infection of pressure injuries due to incontinence. It also allows the ICU staff to collect and analyze the patient's urine.

Additionally, the amount of urine a patient creates indicates kidney health. Generally, more than 30 mL of urine production per hour is healthy. With this information, the ICU staff can determine the patient's fluid balance. This is the amount of fluid that has entered the patient subtracted by the amount urinated. Depending on this calculation, more fluids may be given, or medications may be needed to increase urine production. This balance is especially important for those patients with heart or kidney issues.

Infections from a urinary catheter can be deadly. This is called a catheter-associated urinary tract infection (CAUTI). To prevent infection, the catheter is inserted under sterile precautions, and the site where it enters the body is cleaned once per shift or when dirty. Also, it is removed as soon as it is no longer needed.

There are other tools to help manage urine after the catheter is removed. These are called external catheters. For males, a condom catheter can be effective. It looks like a condom with an opening at the tip that drains urine into a bag. There is a different design for females. It is a hollow tube that is attached to low-powered suction and rests along the groin. The tube is covered in soft fabric, which allows urine to be suctioned through it into a container. The nurse can explain about these and other options.

- Who Performs the Procedure
  - A nurse.
- Its Purpose
  - Measuring fluid balance, relieving urinary retention and obstruction, preventing skin breakdown and infection, and obtaining urinary labs.
- Family Participation
  - Although inserted sterilely, family members may stay in the room if they wish.
  - Monitor for redness and discharge at the insertion site or a change in the clarity of the urine.

Figure 4.12 Urinary (Foley) Catheter

The urinary catheter drains the bladder and measures urine production.

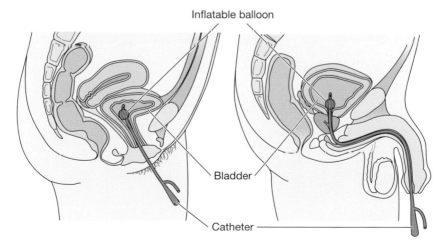

Inflatable balloon

Bladder

Catheter

Sterile Precautions

Sterile precautions are used during some medical procedures. Examples include inserting a urinary catheter or central line. The hardware used in these procedures increases the risk for infection because it is inserted into the body and remains there for days. Germs can then grow on this medical equipment and make their way into the patient. Once inside, an already ill patient now has to fight this infection. The ICU staff takes this very seriously and follows strict rules to prevent it from happening. An important prevention method is using sterile precautions.

During sterile precautions, the family is usually asked to wait outside because only the required staff are allowed in the room. Typically, the patient's skin is disinfected, and sterile gloves are worn. A cloth may be placed over the patient's body with a hole exposing the site where the procedure takes place. The point of this is to clean the skin and prevent germs from reaching the site. After the device has been inserted, the medical team may place a dressing over the site to prevent germs from growing there. The nurse changes the dressing regularly, cleans the area if needed, and watches for signs of infection. Signs of infection include redness, pain, warmth, swelling, or discharge around the device.

5

Medications

Medications are a key part of the care a patient receives in the intensive care unit (ICU). The providers, nurses, and pharmacists team up to provide the best combination of medicine for each patient. Prescribed by a provider after a diagnosis is made, medications are approved or suggested by the pharmacists, and the nurse gives them while monitoring the patient for their effects.

Additionally, with the help of electronic medical records, the administration of medication is safer than ever. It is easy to see how much of each medication the patient has received, and harmful combinations of medicine are flagged to be avoided.

The first step in administering medication is to scan the patient's armband to bring up their medical profile. Next, the medication is scanned to confirm it matches what is prescribed for the patient. If any detail of this process does not match, for instance the wrong medication is scanned, this process will be interrupted, requiring the nurse to examine the prescription more closely. After the medications are confirmed for the patient, the nurse administers them.

A fundamental element of the nurse's job is to follow the "six rights" of medication administration: the right patient is receiving the medication, the right medication for the patient, the right route to administer it (meaning through the IV, swallowing, etc), the right time for it to be administered, the right dose of the medication, and the right effect of the medicine.

Nurse's Note

- If you do not know what medication you are taking, ask the nurse.
- By keeping track of the medications and whether they are having the right effect, you can be another "right" for the patient.
- Do not take your medications, supplements, or vitamins from outside the hospital without asking the nurse first. The medical team keeps track of everything, and many vitamins or supplements do not mix well with hospital medications.
- Let the nurse know if you are not getting the medications that you usually take outside of the hospital.

Medication Timing

Knowing the scheduling of medicine is important for patients and families. Usually, it is ordered in timed segments. For instance, Tylenol, the brand name for acetaminophen, can be ordered to be given every 6 hours. So, the patient receives it at 6 AM, 12 noon, 6 PM, and midnight. Nurses have some wiggle room in when they can administer the medicine. They have about an hour before and after the medication is scheduled to give it. For example, if it is scheduled at 6 AM, it can be given from 5 to 7 AM. This range can differ depending on the hospital.

Another type of order is called a PRN, Latin for "as needed." These medications can only be used in specific situations. For instance, the order may say that it can only be administered if the patient is experiencing breakthrough pain—pain that surges even though it should be under control by the scheduled meds. The instructions may be "give for pain greater than 7 out of 10, every 6 hours." Therefore, nurses can give that med for greater than 7 out of 10 pain at 6:00 AM, but then cannot give it again until noon. It helps to be familiar with these rules so the patient can know when to expect medications that are already ordered and decide if extra medication needs to be prescribed.

Nurse's Note

- If you notice that you received a helpful medication earlier and then not again (eg, cough medicine, eye drops, sleep aid, nicotine patch, pain medication), it may be ordered PRN. Ask the nurse if it is still available or if the provider can order it again.

Pain

Many ICU patients experience pain. Pain medicine, or analgesic, can help to reduce the pain. Frustratingly, there is a limit to what pain medicine can do. After an operation, accident, or illness, there still can be pain and discomfort no matter how much analgesic is given. So, the ICU staff tries to lower the pain to a tolerable level that allows the patient to work at recovering.

For example, eliminating all discomfort following broken ribs is rare. If pain is preventing these patients from breathing effectively, they will not be able to get out of bed and move around—an important part of recovery. Pain also disrupts sleep, hunger, and mood, and these problems result in worse healing. Thus, enough pain control is needed to recover and avoid complications from the injury.

Problematically, too much pain medicine can cause drowsiness and a reduction in actively recovering. For instance, an overmedicated patient can feel less motivated to work with the physical therapist or may be unable to safely participate in swallowing practice with the speech therapist. Therefore, the best goal is to use the least amount of medicine to make the pain tolerable. Too much pain sidelines the patient. Too much pain medicine slows recovery.

Each patient's pain tolerance is different. A 95-year-old woman may barely flinch when a chest tube is pulled from her lung. Also, a 30-year-old man may agonize as a piece of tape is pulled off his hand. Both of these reactions are equally valid, and care is taken to support each individual's needs.

To do this, the ICU staff asks the patient for a pain goal that is acceptable, realistic, and allows for participation in recovery. Thankfully, the caregivers and patients have many ways to work together to find that sweet spot.

For patients who can communicate, pain usually is assessed on a 0 to 10 scale, where 0 is no pain and 10 is the worst possible. It helps to add descriptions, such as aching, stabbing, throbbing, etc, and where the pain is felt. In addition, try to remember when it started and note if anything makes it better or worse. With this information, caregivers can get a better idea of what is bothering the patient, what may help best, and compare it to pain felt later.

Nurse's Note

■ Providing details about your pain allows the medical team to treat it better. A helpful way to describe your symptoms is to remember the letters of the alphabet OPQRST.

■ Onset—When did your pain start?

■ Provokes—What makes your pain worse?

■ Qualities—What does your pain feel like?

■ Region—Where is your pain?

■ Severity—How bad is your pain on a 0 to 10 scale?

■ Treatment—Has anything helped your pain?

Other tools are used to help the ICU staff rate pain for patients who cannot communicate. For these patients, caregivers can assess grimacing, moaning, and other clues that indicate discomfort. By comparing those signs before and after pain medicine is given, the ICU staff can see if that medicine is effective.

The goal is to reduce the pain to a tolerable level as soon as possible. However, effectively managing pain does not happen immediately. Pain medications take time to work, and they do not work for all patients. Other ways to reduce pain without medicine, such as ice and heat, also have to be tried. The medical staff thanks all patients for working through this challenging process.

Nurse's Note

■ Pain tolerance is a personal experience for the patient that can change in different settings. The pain a patient feels now is true and valid, even if it seems like it should not be "that" painful. Additionally, patients may act fine, but say their pain is terrible. It is important that the medical team and family support patients in both of these scenarios because the patients are the only ones who truly know the pain they are experiencing. If you respond to how your loved one is, not how you expect your loved one to be, they feel supported and are more likely to work to get better.

■ Think about whether the pain you are experiencing is a new pain that recently started (acute) or a pain that you have experienced for a while (chronic). If it is a chronic pain (for example, lower back pain you have had for years), tell the nurse if anything helps relieve the pain at home. Those options, or similar ones, may be available in the hospital.

Managing Pain Without Medicine

There are many ways to reduce pain without medication, and the ICU staff uses these as much as possible. These options may be called nonpharmacological pain management. They have few side effects and can help reduce the amount of pain medicine that is needed.

Spending time in bed can cause muscle aches. Heat can be used to soothe an achy back or neck. It helps loosen up muscles that are sore or tight. It is great before physical therapy to get the patient ready to move.

Ice helps numb pain and reduce any swelling. Patients with recent injuries or surgeries can benefit from icing swollen or painful areas. Ice may be especially useful after activity to reduce any nagging pain. Additionally, it can help reduce a headache.

Changing position in bed helps relieve pressure on the body. If possible, getting out of bed for a walk or into the chair can feel even better. It helps get the blood moving, exercises the lung and muscles, and gives the patient a sense of accomplishment. If a patient had a chest surgery, a technique called splinting can reduce pain during movement. The patient holds a pillow to their chest while coughing or moving.

Distraction is another effective tool. The family can help by making the patient think about other things besides pain. For instance, playing music or watching a movie can help pass the time. Talking to the patient about their day, remembering positive experiences such as vacations or time outside of the hospital, or even a massage can take their mind off of the pain. Another type of distraction is acupressure, which makes the patient feel the part of the body being touched more than the pain. Focusing on breathing and mindfulness can also reduce pain sensation, and there are many phone apps to help practice this. The family is welcome to suggest other options to help with pain control.

Each option helps time pass until the next pain medication is needed. Although it is OK to take pain medicine if necessary, it is better to help the patient heal with the least amount possible. If the amount of medicine is reduced, the patient is less likely to have bad side effects.

Nurse's Note

- Encourage the patient to try these types of pain control.
- Ask the nurse to show you safe ways to massage and perform acupressure, and if other medication-free ways to reduce pain can be used.

Pain Medicine

There are multiple types of pain medicine that are commonly used in the ICU. Usually, patients think of opioids as the answer for pain. Examples include fentanyl, oxycodone, morphine, and hydromorphone. Although safe and effective for intense pain, they can create other issues.

Opioids can cause constipation, drowsiness, nausea, and increase the risk of aspiration. They also can reduce the drive to breathe and lower blood pressure, which can be a problem for those patients who already have breathing or blood pressure issues. Worryingly, they can cause dependence and addiction if used for extended periods. Because of these reasons, the ICU staff tries to use the least amount of opioids possible to make pain manageable. To help achieve this goal, other non-opioid pain medicines are given for additional relief. This strategy is called multimodal pain management.

Nurse's Note

- Because many patients are constipated due to surgery or opioids, intense gas pains can result that are distressing. A medicine called simethicone can provide relief.
- If you use opioids at home, let the ICU team know. This helps the ICU team develop a better pain management plan for you.

To reduce the amount of opioids needed, acetaminophen is commonly prescribed. When used with opioids, the total amount of pain medicine needed is usually decreased. Acetaminophen is helpful for many types of pain, including headaches and soreness accompanying surgeries, and for lowering fevers. This medicine may be avoided for those with liver injury, as it can cause liver damage.

Nurse's Note

■ IV acetaminophen can be helpful if you are in severe pain and want to reduce your opioid use.

Other non-opioid pain relievers are ibuprofen and ketorolac. These are a type of medication called a nonsteroidal anti-inflammatory drug (NSAID), and they reduce inflammation and pain. Although effective, they are given less frequently than acetaminophen because they can cause stomach bleeding and kidney damage.

Another way to reduce pain is a lidocaine patch. This sticky pad is left on for 12 hours and numbs the area where it is placed. Lidocaine works best for muscle aches and pain felt just below the skin.

Nurse's Note

■ If moving hurts, taking pain medicine before working with physical therapy (PT) and occupational therapy (OT) can help the patient have more effective therapy. This is called premedicating. Take oral medications about an hour before and IV medications about 10 minutes before the activity.

■ Take note of how different pain medications make you feel. For example, if IV opioids make you sleepy, they may not be the best choice for pain control before PT. Your nurse can help make a plan for you.

■ Some hospitals have a pain service that specializes in helping patients with complicated pain issues. If pain has not been adequately controlled, ask if the pain service is available for consult. Importantly, give the ICU team time to find the right strategy for your pain management.

Patient-Controlled Analgesia: Patient-Controlled Pain Medicine

If a patient has intense pain for a long time, or is returning from surgery, the ICU team may use another tool in addition to scheduled and PRN pain medicine. Some hospitals use a medication pump that allows for patient-controlled analgesia (PCA). This can be programmed to deliver IV pain medicine continuously or on-demand, or both. If on-demand, the nurse gives the patient a button to press that can deliver the medicine about every 10 minutes. This allows patients to decide when they are in too much pain and helps to relieve anxiety about pain control. The PCA is set to a maximum amount of medication that can be given in an hour, and the medical team can increase this if it is not enough.

A similar tool for pain relief is the epidural PCA, which eases pain only in one area of the body. A tiny tube is placed in the back by the spine, and pain medicine flows through this. Similar to how the pain of labor is reduced during pregnancy, this blocks pain in specific areas. For instance, a patient may only have pain in the legs, which could be controlled with an epidural. This option is typically used after an operation, when it is known where pain control will be important.

Nurse's Note

- The epidural PCA, and opioids in general, may cause itching, which can be reduced with medicine.
- Only the patient should press the button for pain medicine.

Figure 5.1 Patient-Controlled Analgesia

Patient-controlled analgesia is a tool for pain management. Pain medicine is delivered when the button is pressed. It may reduce the anxiety of pain control and reduce the amount of pain medicine needed.

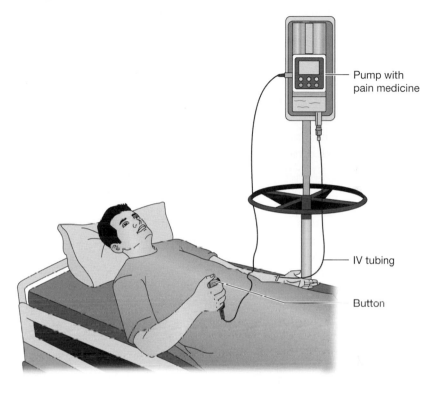

Pump with pain medicine

IV tubing

Button

Vasoactive Medications: Controlling Blood Pressure

Vasoactive medications are used to increase or decrease blood pressure. They allow the ICU staff to lower dangerously high blood pressure (hypertension) to prevent bleeding and organ damage. Or, these medications can raise dangerously low blood pressure (hypotension) to help blood reach the patient's organs. These medications are given continuously by medication pumps, and the amount given is adjusted by the nurse. These medications save lives.

The vasoactive medications that decrease blood pressure work by slowing the heart rate or widening (dilating) the blood vessels. Examples of these medications are nicardipine and nitroglycerin. These types of medicine are commonly used to prevent the dangerous effects of high blood pressure, such as bleeding in the brain. They are also common after surgery. The ICU staff keeps the patient's blood pressure in a narrow range to prevent the new, fragile incision from being forced open by high blood pressure.

If blood pressure is too low, the patient's organs do not receive the oxygen needed to function. This damages the organs and can cause death. To raise blood pressure, vasoactive medications narrow (constrict) blood vessels or increase the ability of the heart to pump blood. These medications can also be called vasopressors, or pressors. Examples of vasopressors include norepinephrine and dopamine. They are used for very sick patients and require a central line to administer them safely. An arterial line is preferred when using these medications because it provides a real-time blood pressure reading. This indicates to the ICU staff if more or less of the vasopressor is needed to reach the right blood pressure.

Generally, the blood pressure goal is to keep the patient's mean arterial pressure (MAP, the number to the right of the top and bottom blood pressure numbers) greater than 65. This is the pressure needed to deliver blood to the organs. If the MAP stays below 65, more of the vasopressor is given. However, there is a maximum amount that is effective, and another vasopressor may be added if the limit of the first is reached. Sadly, the patient's chance of recovery becomes worse when more vasopressors are needed. As patients get better, they are slowly taken off of these medications one at a time, so long as the MAP is greater than 65.

Sedation: Calming the Patient

Patients can experience anxiety and distress from their illness, being in the ICU, and treatments needed to make them better. Sedation medication not only helps calm patients, but it also allows the ICU therapies to work more effectively.

Which medication the staff uses depends on what level of sedation the patient needs. The levels are mild, moderate, deep, and general. General sedation is only used in the operating room, so the highest level experienced in the ICU is deep sedation.

Mild Sedation: Reducing Anxiety

Mild sedation is used for anxious patients. The ICU staff tries all other relaxation strategies before medication is used. Depending on what is causing the distress, these patients are usually given anti-anxiety medicine or pain medicine to relax them.

Nurse's Note

- Family is very helpful in calming anxious patients. Focusing on breathing, tidying up their space, supporting the patient by saying "you are doing a good job," massages, music, conversation, pictures, holding a hand, video games, phone calls, etc, are all welcome.
- Encourage your loved one to focus on doing things that make them better. For instance, use the incentive spirometer, do some of the exercises PT or OT left for the patient, ask the nurse to walk, etc.
- Let the nurse know if you take anything for anxiety at home, or what usually helps with your anxiety.
- If you use tobacco, let the nurse know. A nicotine patch may help with anxiety.

Moderate Sedation: Relaxing the Patient During a Procedure

During painful or uncomfortable procedures, such as a bronchoscopy, a moderate level of sedation is best. This may also be called conscious sedation.

Different medications can accomplish moderate sedation. A common combination of medications is an opioid, usually fentanyl, to reduce pain, and a benzodiazepine, usually midazolam, to prevent memories of the event and anxiety. Patients are able to breathe on their own, but emergency equipment is available just in case it is needed. The medical team keeps a close eye on the patient and their vital signs during and after the procedure.

Nurse's Note

- Some of these procedures are sterile or uncomfortable to watch, so family may be asked to wait outside.
- The patient should return to how they were acting preprocedure within about an hour.

Deep Sedation: Relaxation During Extended Therapy

Deep sedation can be used for many critical illnesses, such as a patient with serious brain, heart, or lung problems. Because these problems reduce the patient's ability to breathe, a breathing tube is needed. The combination of this tube, the help provided by the breathing machine (ventilator), and the therapies needed to treat these illnesses can be uncomfortable. Deep sedation makes these tolerable by relaxing the patient and reducing the ability to remember the experience. A commonly used medication to achieve deep sedation is propofol. It should be noted that propofol does not prevent pain. So, if the patient is in distress, pain medicine may need to be given.

Depending on the reason for deep sedation, patients can usually still respond in a sleepy way to the caregivers. The medical team uses the least amount of sedation to make the patient comfortable and allow the therapies to work. Too much sedation can cause the patient to have low blood pressure and spend a longer time in the ICU. Please see Sedation, page 92, for details about reducing and turning off the sedation.

Nurse's Note

■ Some patients say they can hear what is happening around them under deep sedation. These patients enjoy their families talking to them, holding a hand, listening to music, etc, during these times. Be sure to check with the nurse to make sure it is OK.

Dexmedetomidine is a mild sedative that is useful in many scenarios. It reduces anxiety and does not decrease the ability to breathe. Patients can be awake and responsive while on this medication. Therefore, it can be given to patients without breathing tubes. Also, when added to the medications needed for deep sedation, it lowers the amount of other sedatives needed. However, it can decrease blood pressure and heart rate. The medical team keeps a close eye on the effects that these medications are having and adjusts them if necessary.

Ketamine is a medication that is used for both deep sedation and pain relief. It has no negative effect on breathing or blood pressure, but it can cause hallucinogenic experiences at high levels. The ICU staff tries to minimize these by using the least amount of medication necessary. Combining ketamine with other sedatives can lower the total amount of sedation medication needed by the patient.

Paralytic: Preventing Patients From Working Against Themselves

ICU patients sometimes work against the therapies that are helping to save their lives. Although the patients are not doing it on purpose, the ICU staff needs to prevent them from disrupting their treatment. The best way to help these patients is by using medication that temporarily paralyzes them. This is reversible, and it can save lives.

For instance, patients can prevent the ventilator from giving enough air by coughing or trying to breathe on their own. This is known as fighting, or being dyssynchronous, with the ventilator. This makes the therapy less effective. After the patient is temporarily paralyzed, the uninterrupted ventilator is able to give the right amount of air to open the patient's lungs.

The first step is to bring the patient under deep sedation. This is to make sure that they are unaware of the temporary paralyzation. A paralytic medication, such as cisatracurium, is then infused. The patient is not given too much because this can weaken their muscles and make their ICU stay longer. Usually after 48 hours, the paralytic is stopped, and it naturally wears off. If safe for the patient, the sedation can then be reduced.

To make sure the right amount of medication is given for paralysis and sedation, two tools are used. The first is bispectral index monitoring (BIS). This measures the patient's brain waves to make sure they are not aware of the paralyzation. The BIS number matches the amount of the patient's brain activity. As the patient goes into deeper sedation, the BIS number decreases because there is less brain activity. An awake patient has a BIS number near 100, while the goal for sedation is around 40 to 60. The nurse adjusts the amount of sedation given until the patient is in this range.

The other tool, train of four, measures the paralytic's effect on the patient by sending four small electrical pulses through face, hand, or ankle nerves. In a patient with no paralytic, these shocks cause four small muscle twitches. As more medication is given, fewer twitches occur. The goal is usually two or three twitches. The nurse adjusts the amount of paralytic to achieve this goal.

Figure 5.2 Bispectral Index Monitor

The bispectral index monitor measures the patient's brain activity. Typically, it is used when giving both sedating and paralyzing medications.

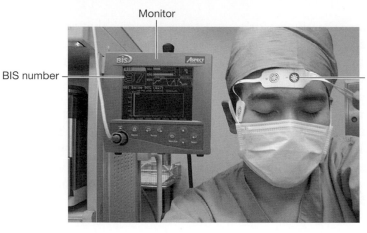

Figure 5.3 Train of Four

The train of four measures the patient's response to paralyzing medication. The electrodes can be placed on the forearm, brow, or ankle.

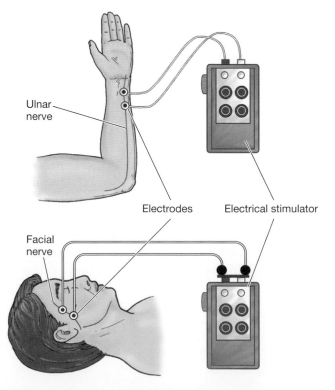

6

Lab Tests
How to Understand the Patient's Labs

All intensive care units (ICUs) use blood for testing, and these laboratory tests are called labs or blood work. Labs are one of the most important tools available to tell how the patient is doing. At a minimum, labs are taken each night. About 1 tablespoon of blood is needed for the 2 standard tests, a complete blood count (CBC) and a basic metabolic panel (BMP). The CBC tells how many of each type of blood cell are present. The BMP shows the kidney function, blood sugar, and amount of electrolytes present. If the patient is unstable or has certain conditions, these labs and others are taken more frequently.

Nurse's Note

- If the medical team has to repeatedly poke you or your loved one to draw blood, it may be best to request a more dependable (and less painful) way to draw blood, such as a peripherally inserted central catheter (PICC).
- Let the nurse know if there is a spot that is usually the best to draw blood.
- The more hydrated a patient is, the easier it is to draw blood. Also, it is helpful if the patient flexes their muscles and warms the area where they will be poked.

What the Labs Can Tell About the Patient

This section explains which labs are important for different illnesses. The patient's blood gives clues about what is going on in their body. By tracking the hints that the blood samples provide, the ICU staff can tell the direction a patient's condition is heading.

Keep in mind, one lab value taken at one time cannot tell if the patient is getting better or worse. The team looks at all of the labs, medications, images, and the other patient symptoms over time to develop a full picture. To do this, many of the same labs are repeated to see how the illness is progressing.

The following is a guide to the clues given by blood work. This also gives an idea of what the ICU staff looks for in the lab results. Importantly, there are many conditions that can alter the labs mentioned, and there are different interpretations for the same lab result. This is a general guide so patients and families can know which labs may be important to follow for the patient's specific illness.

Nurse's Note

- Always compare the current labs to what they were and reflect on what happened to the patient in between each test.
- Normal levels can vary between each person, so it is important to compare the labs to the patient's usual values.

Illnesses and Their Labs

Bleeding

- Hemoglobin
  - The part of blood that carries oxygen and carbon dioxide.
  - A lower result can indicate bleeding.
  - Receiving fluids can dilute the amount of hemoglobin, making it look falsely low (dilutional).
  - Part of the CBC.
- Hematocrit
  - Percentage of red blood cells in the blood.
  - A lower result can indicate bleeding.

- This can be diluted with fluids, making it look falsely low.
- Part of the CBC.
- Platelets
  - The body's way of stopping a bleed.
  - A lower result means the patient is at risk for bleeding more easily.
  - Can be lower due to infections.
  - Part of the CBC.
- Prothrombin Time (PT)
  - The amount of time blood takes to begin clotting.
  - A higher number means it takes longer to clot, and therefore the patient can bleed more easily.
- International Normalized Ratio (INR)
  - A measure of how fast the patient's blood clots compared to normal.
  - A higher number means it takes longer to clot, and therefore the patient can bleed more easily.
  - Can be used to evaluate a patient's response to warfarin, a blood thinner.
- Partial Thromboplastin Time (PTT)
  - The amount of time blood takes to begin clotting.
  - A higher number means it takes longer to clot, and therefore the patient can bleed more easily.
  - Can be used to evaluate a patient's response to heparin, a blood thinner.
  - This lab is taken every six hours if the patient is receiving heparin continuously. The ICU staff uses the PTT number to see if more or less heparin is needed.

Infection

- White Blood Cells (WBCs)
  - How the body fights infections.
  - A higher number can mean the body is fighting an infection.
  - If the amount of WBCs is high, the ICU staff try to find if an infection is present in the blood or other body fluids (cultures).
  - Part of the CBC.
- Cultures
  - Indicates if an infection is present where the sample was collected.
  - Can test blood, urine, sputum (from the lungs), a wound, or other bodily fluids.
  - Takes more than 24 hours to show if germs are present.
  - Tells which medicine can kill the infection.

Kidney Injury

- Creatinine
  - A substance that is removed from the blood by the kidneys.
  - A higher amount of it can indicate worse kidney function.
  - Part of the BMP.
- Electrolytes
  - Minerals that allow the body to function.
    - Some examples are potassium, magnesium, and calcium.
  - Levels are regulated by the kidneys.
  - Low and high levels can cause irregular heartbeats.
  - The ICU staff may give patients electrolytes if they are low.
  - The ICU staff treats high levels with medicine and may recommend dialysis (using a machine to filter out the electrolytes).
  - Part of the BMP.

Liver Injury

- Aspartate Transaminase (AST)
  - A substance, called an enzyme, found in the liver.
  - A higher amount can indicate liver damage.
- Alanine Transaminase (ALT)
  - A substance, called an enzyme, found in the liver.
  - A higher amount can indicate liver damage.
- Bilirubin
  - A chemical that is produced after red blood cells are broken down.
  - A higher amount can indicate liver damage.

Heart Injury

- Troponin
  - A chemical released from the heart if it is damaged.
  - A higher amount can mean heart stress or injury.
  - Usually measured if a heart attack is suspected.
  - If the amount of this chemical is higher than normal, it is usually monitored every few hours until it decreases. If it gets higher, this can mean new damage is occurring.
- B-Type Natriuretic Peptide (BNP)
  - A chemical that is elevated when the chambers of the heart are filled with too much blood.
  - A higher amount can indicate heart failure.

Diabetes

- Hemoglobin A1C
  - A chemical that indicates the level of sugar in the blood over the last 3 months.
  - An elevated level increases the chance of developing diabetes.
  - Multiple elevated levels show the patient has diabetes.
  - High levels increase the risk for negative effects of diabetes.

Other Labs

- Lactate
  - A chemical that is produced when tissues do not get oxygen.
  - An elevated level indicates less oxygen is in the tissues.
  - Can be high because of low blood pressure or infection.
- Arterial Blood Gas
  - A complex lab that can mean many things.
  - Measures how well the lungs and kidneys are working.
  - Indicates how much oxygen the patient has in their blood.
    - Normal oxygen level is 80 to 100.
  - Indicates how much carbon dioxide the patient has in their blood.
    - Normal carbon dioxide level is 35 to 45.

7

Possible Side Effects of the ICU

Delirium, Restraints, and Pressure Injuries

Delirium: When the Patient Becomes Confused

It can be hard for patients to maintain a clear and focused mind in the intensive care unit (ICU). Pain, the experience of the illness, stress from the therapies, and the unfamiliar environment can make the patient's mind hazy. Furthermore, sleep is frequently interrupted, and it can be hard to remember the date and time as days blend together. To make things worse, sedatives and opioids can cause confusion. These disturbances can all result in a condition called <u>delirium</u>, which many patients experience in the ICU.

Delirium is a sudden change in mental sharpness (the patient's ability to understand where they are and what is going on), a reduced awareness of surroundings, and a decreased ability to focus, speak, think, or remember. A patient's behavior can also change, either by becoming more active (restless or agitated), less active (sleepy or in a daze), or alternating between the two. Patients can become delirious within a day or two of being in the ICU. It is most common at night, and the level of delirium usually changes throughout the day. For instance, a patient may be delirious overnight, but return to a normal state of mind in the morning.

Nurse's Note

■ Let the medical team know immediately if your family member is acting differently. The medical team may ask you to describe how they usually behave.

■ Another reason for a sudden change in a patient's behavior may be a brain injury, called a stroke. Please see the Code Stroke section for the common signs of a stroke (page 129).

■ Delirium and dementia are often confused. Delirium changes over the course of the day and is a quick change. Dementia is a less sudden change in abilities that starts small and gradually gets worse. Sometimes the only way to tell the difference is by asking the patient to focus on a task. The delirious patient has trouble concentrating, while the patient with dementia can attempt to focus on the task. It is also possible for a patient to have delirium and dementia.

Among all the stressful side effects of the ICU, delirium can be the most disturbing for family members. Seemingly without a cause, patients can become panicked, confused, or "out of it." They can also have trouble remembering details, see things that are not there, or repeat pointless movements.

Delirium usually improves as the patient gets healthier. Worryingly, it can take a while to fully regain their mental abilities, and delirium may cause permanent harm to the brain. Because of this, preventing, recognizing, and treating the causes of delirium quickly are important.

Preventing delirium starts with encouraging activity throughout the day and making nights as restful as possible. At all times, hearing and visual aids should be easily accessible for the patient. Discomforts, such as pain, thirst, hunger, anxiety, and needing to use the restroom should be addressed quickly. Furthermore, the medical team and family can work together to reduce the need for medications that increase the risk for delirium. For instance, effectively managing pain with minimal opioid medication is one way to help. Another way to prevent delirium is to reduce stress by creating a soothing and familiar environment.

Nurse's Note

- Delirium can be caused by many things. Sometimes, simply the change of environment can begin this condition. If your loved one becomes delirious, do not blame yourself. It is not your fault.

The medical team continually looks for any signs of delirium. They frequently test reasoning, memory, and mental sharpness through conversation and by asking patients their name, the date, and where they are. If confused, the medical team reorients the patient (reminds them of where they are, the date, etc) and tries to limit any potential causes of delirium.

Nurse's Note

- Help reorient patients by telling them where they are, the date and time, how long they have been there, how they got there, what happened during the day, what is happening tomorrow, etc.
- Bring pictures from home to make the room more familiar.
- Open the blinds and turn on the lights during the day. Exercise however possible (physical therapy and occupational therapy can provide suggestions).
- At night, close the blinds, turn off the TV, and help create a good sleeping environment. If the patient has before-bed habits, family members can help them through their nighttime routine. Sleep aids, such as melatonin, can help the patient sleep without causing delirium. Ear plugs and eye masks may also be available.
- You can ask the medical team to try to allow the patient to sleep through the night with minimal disturbances. If your loved one is very ill, this may not be possible.
- If the patient is delirious but allowed to eat or drink, make sure the patient is totally awake, sitting up straight, and monitored closely. Do not leave food and drink close by without supervision.
- Mention if your loved one has had delirium before or if they drink alcohol, use drugs, or are taking anything at home for pain or anxiety.
- Please visit NavigatingTheICU.com for more resources.

Figure 7.1 The Confusion Assessment Method for the ICU

The Confusion Assessment Method for the ICU (CAM-ICU) is one of the tools used to assess for delirium. For step 3, a patient with a RASS of zero is calm and awake. A patient who is more active or less active than normal is not a RASS of zero.

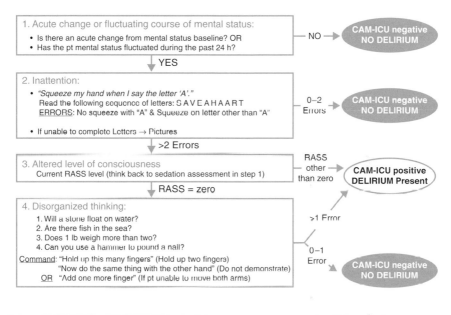

DELIRIUM ASSESSMENT

1. Acute change or fluctuating course of mental status:
   - Is there an acute change from mental status baseline? OR
   - Has the pt mental status fluctuated during the past 24 h?

NO → CAM-ICU negative NO DELIRIUM

↓ YES

2. Inattention:
   - *"Squeeze my hand when I say the letter 'A'."*
     Read the following sequence of letters: S A V E A H A A R T
     <u>ERRORS</u>: No squeeze with "A" & Squeeze on letter other than "A"
   - If unable to complete Letters → Pictures

0–2 Errors → CAM-ICU negative NO DELIRIUM

↓ >2 Errors

3. Altered level of consciousness
   Current RASS level (think back to sedation assessment in step 1)

RASS other than zero → CAM-ICU positive DELIRIUM Present

↓ RASS = zero

4. Disorganized thinking:
   1. Will a stone float on water?
   2. Are there fish in the sea?
   3. Does 1 lb weigh more than two?
   4. Can you use a hammer to pound a nail?
   <u>Command</u>: "Hold up this many fingers" (Hold up two fingers)
   "Now do the same thing with the other hand" (Do not demonstrate)
   <u>OR</u> "Add one more finger" (If pt unable to move both arms)

>1 Error

0–1 Error → CAM-ICU negative NO DELIRIUM

Restraints: Restraining Movement for Safety

Because patients can be confused in the ICU, their movement may have to be restricted for their safety. Using <u>restraints</u> is a last resort, but unfortunately is a necessary part of the ICU. There are strict rules for when they may be used, as well as when they need to be removed. Additionally, the documentation of restraints is closely monitored to make sure they are being used appropriately and safely.

The most common use for restraints is when a patient needs the breathing tube. The tube is uncomfortable, and many patients instinctively try to pull it out. Unfortunately, this happens and is very scary. The patient removes the tube before being able to breathe on their own. This is an emergency, and the tube needs to be replaced quickly or the patient may die. Therefore, to protect the patient, wrist restraints are used until the medical staff remove the breathing tube. They are soft cuffs that go around the patient's wrists and are tied to the bed. They limit the movement of the arms so the patient cannot reach the breathing tube.

The fundamental reason restraints are used is that patients can become a danger to themselves. Examples of this include pulling out medical equipment, such as the breathing tube, or risking a fall by trying to unsafely get out of bed. This behavior can be caused by many things, including the illness, delirium, dementia, or drug withdrawal. Importantly, not all people in those categories are restrained, only those who may be hurt by their actions. Additionally, the ICU staff tries other strategies to limit this behavior before restraints are used. For instance, if a patient is unsafely trying to get out of bed, the nurse can use the help of a patient-care technician to watch the patient or set the bed alarm to notify everyone when the patient is trying to get up. Only after these and other measures fail are restraints used.

Restraints may also be needed if a patient needs medication to support their blood pressure, but they are attempting to pull out their IV. The lines can be hidden or taped down, but if the patient continues to pull them, restraints are necessary. Importantly, if the patient is capable of making decisions about their treatment, the medical care can be refused. Restraints are reserved for those people who lack the capacity to make decisions and are a danger to their own health.

The least restrictive restraints necessary are used to stop the harmful activity. Wrist restraints usually are the first line. Another option are mittens that cover the hands so a patient cannot pick at things. If patients are flailing their legs, ankle restraints that secure the ankles to the bed can be used. Very agitated patients can be tied to the bed with a chest strap.

Patients who are spitting, kicking, punching, etc, are classified as violent. This is another category of restrained patient. Attempts are made to calm the patient as much as possible. Sometimes a medical team that specializes in these situations can be called to help the patient.

Medical care is still provided to all patients. Nursing duties, such as administering medication, examining the patient, toileting, feeding, etc, continue even when patients become violent. Nurses are also careful that the restraints do not cause injuries. Once the unsafe behavior has ended, these devices are removed.

Nurse's Note

- Help soothe the patient and encourage them to not remove medical equipment.
- Please let the nurse know if your loved one is being unsafe (trying to get out of bed, pulling on things, etc)—if something is bothering them, the nurse may be able to hide it or give them a break from it.

Figure 7.2 Mitten Restraints

Mittens may be necessary for unsafe patients who repeatedly remove equipment.

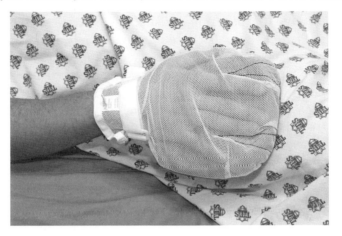

Figure 7.3 Wrist Restraints

Wrist restraints may be necessary for unsafe patients who repeatedly try to get out of bed or remove equipment. They are secured to the bed with a quick-release knot.

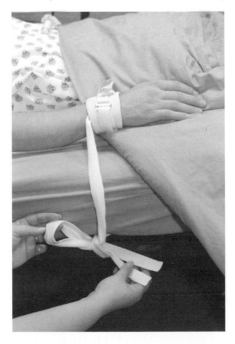

Pressure Injuries: Skin Breakdown From Pressure

Patients in the ICU have a high risk for skin injuries. Their skin is more fragile than usual because they are usually eating and drinking less, they are attached to medical equipment, and their skin becomes dry. Also, blood flow to the skin decreases with less exercise or low blood pressure.

When skin is pinched between the patient's bone and an object, the supply of blood flow stops. Eventually, this soft tissue dies. This is known as a <u>pressure injury</u> (PI), bedsore, or pressure ulcer. If fat or muscle is also squeezed, it can die as well.

ICU patients spend many hours in bed, making this surface a common cause of pressure. PIs are usually found where the bed meets bony areas, such as the tailbone, hips, spine, heels, or back of the head. Additionally, medical equipment, such as the feeding tube or wires, can also cause a PI.

The ICU staff try to prevent a PI from developing. Foam pads are used to cover bony areas that commonly pinch the skin, and frequent skin assessments are required. If possible, medical devices are padded, changed positions to reduce pressure to any one area of the skin, and monitored regularly for evidence of skin breakdown. Nurses shift the patient's weight every 2 hours while in bed to avoid prolonged pressure. Pillows can be used to lift the heels and elbows off the mattress. Nutrition, getting the patient out of bed, and exercise are started as soon as possible.

Moisture from incontinence can also weaken the skin, making a PI morel likely. Ways to limit this include reducing skin contact with moisture by using internal or external urinary catheters, gently cleaning the skin with cleanser after incontinence, and applying cream to shield the skin from bodily fluids.

It only takes about 2 hours of constant pressure for a PI to form. If the pressure continues, it can get worse. A PI can range from stage 1 to stage 4:

Stage 1: A red or discolored spot on the skin (epidermis) that does not get whiter when pressed.
Stage 2: A blister or break in the skin.
Stage 3: Fat tissue exposed without bone or muscle visible.
Stage 4: Bone or muscle exposed.

Once a PI is noticed, the ICU team provides care for the wound. There may be a nurse who specializes in identifying wounds and providing treatment. This nurse assesses the injury, recommends the best way to care for it, and regularly revisits to see how it is progressing. Special care is provided for these injuries because they heal slowly and can become infected.

Nurse's Note

- Let the nurse know if you see any red or discolored skin, or if the patient is lying on medical equipment.
- If incontinence is occurring, ask the nurse for an external catheter and barrier cream to help protect the skin from breakdown.
- Ask the nurse if you can apply lotion to your loved one, but do so gently.
- Encourage the patient to shift their weight in bed.
- Encourage the patient to exercise with physical therapy and occupational therapy.

Figure 7.4 Pressure Injury Stages

The different stages of a pressure injury depend on the damaged tissue. There can be other types, such as a deep tissue injury, which the nurse or wound care nurse can identify.

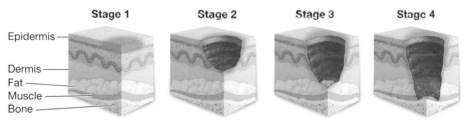

Figure 7.5 Common Pressure Injury Sites

There are many places where pressure injuries can occur, but they are most common over bony areas. Padding these areas and changing positions help prevent these injuries.

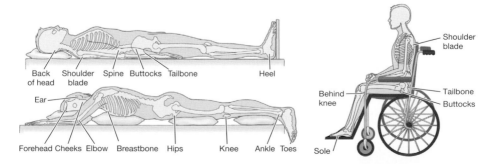

8

Therapies for Common Issues

Helping the Patient's Temperature, Kidneys, and Breathing

Temperature

Cooling the Patient

Patients can develop a fever for different reasons. Usually, it helps the body fight an infection and is healthy. Brain injury and some medications may also cause a fever. If the temperature is too high, it can have negative effects. For instance, a fever can raise the heart rate and stress the heart and lungs. If it is very high, brain damage can occur. If the patient gets too hot, the intensive care unit (ICU) staff uses different tools to lower the temperature.

Depending on the ICU, a fever usually is treated when it rises above 101°F. Acetaminophen, or Tylenol, has fever-reducing properties, and may be all that is needed. Ice packs and cool towels can also work well, especially if placed near arteries in the neck, armpits, or groin. The nurse may also sponge cool water onto the patient.

When a fever is hard to reduce, special tools may be used. One is the cooling blanket, which is a pad with cool water flowing through it. This blanket is placed under or on top of the patient in order to lower their body temperature. Another machine uses cooling pads wrapped around the patient's legs and torso to reduce the temperature. Another option is to cool the body from inside the patient. In this case, a central line with a small balloon is inserted into a vein. The central line is then connected to a cooling machine, which circulates cold fluid fluid through the balloon to reduce the fever. All of these devices are set to a desired temperature and the patient's temperature is monitored continuously.

Nurse's Note

■ Another method for lowering a fever is to leave blankets off of the patient and turn up the air conditioning. Please ask the nurse before adding or removing blankets.

Warming the Patient

Many illnesses decrease blood flow, and this can make patients cold. Additionally, operating rooms are kept cold to prevent the growth of germs. Therefore, patients usually arrive to the ICU chilly after surgery.

Cold patients are warmed by turning up the heat and covering them with warm blankets. A tool called a Bair Hugger is also effective. This is a blanket, laid over the patient, that has warm air circulating through it.

Nurse's Note

■ The Bair Hugger works best with only a sheet over it.

Kidney Damage

Hemodialysis and Continuous Renal Replacement Therapy

The kidneys (renal system) are important for a few reasons. They clean the blood by filtering out any unhealthy waste created by normal bodily functions. This waste leaves the body as urine. The kidneys also keep the right amount of fluid in the body. They sense the fluid levels and, if necessary, change how much urine is made. The kidneys also maintain the right amount of electrolytes in the blood (potassium, magnesium, calcium, etc). The right balance of these minerals is needed for the body to work. The kidneys filter out excess electrolytes into urine. By cleaning the blood, balancing the fluid levels, and maintaining the right amount of electrolytes, the kidneys help the entire body.

Unfortunately, the kidneys can be hurt by many illness and medications. Damage can occur to the kidneys in 3 possible ways: low blood flow to the kidneys (eg, low blood pressure or liver disease), damage to the kidneys themselves (eg, toxic chemicals or COVID-19), or a blockage that prevents urine from leaving the body (eg, enlarged prostate or kidney stones).

When something causes new damage to the kidneys, it is called an acute kidney injury (AKI) or kidney failure. After an AKI, the kidneys do not function as well. Waste, fluid, and electrolytes build up in the body because they cannot be filtered into urine. Eventually, this buildup interferes with the body's ability to work normally. For instance, the increase in potassium in the blood can stop the heart. Another problem occurs when more fluid stays in the body. The body swells and breathing becomes harder and harder. These patients are "fluid overloaded." To help prevent these problems, the ICU team tracks kidney function.

Kidney function is measured by the amount of urine produced and the level of creatinine in the blood (a bodily waste that is removed by the kidneys). If creatinine rises and urine decreases, an AKI usually is the cause. The ICU team then tries to reverse the reason for the AKI. Hopefully, this prevents lasting kidney damage. If the damage is bad enough, the ICU team will recommend dialysis.

Dialysis, or hemodialysis (HD), is a machine that acts like a kidney. It cleans the patient's blood, removes fluid, and balances their electrolytes. It is scheduled usually 3 times per week and lasts about 3 hours. Unfortunately, HD can cause dangerously low blood pressure. If the patient already has issues with low blood pressure, the team may choose continuous renal replacement therapy (CRRT). Both HD and CRRT act like a kidney, but CRRT is a gentler form of HD. Once CRRT starts, it runs continuously. However, CRRT can still cause low blood pressure. Therefore, it may have to be paused until the blood pressure is fixed.

These machines need their own central lines, which allow for a large amount of blood to flow to and from the machine. The line is inserted in the groin, chest, or neck. A specialized dialysis nurse runs HD, while the ICU nurse runs CRRT. The team tracks the kidney function daily to see if HD or CRRT can be stopped.

Nurse's Note

- If your loved one has a kidney injury, the ICU team may limit how much fluid they can drink. This is to prevent the buildup of fluid in the body. Please see NPO (page 120) for suggestions about how to help relieve thirst.
- Those with kidney injury may have a special diet that is low in salt and electrolytes. This is to reduce the buildup of those minerals in the body.
- Consent is needed for these therapies.

Figure 8.1 Hemodialysis

When the kidneys are seriously injured, dialysis is needed to clean the blood and remove fluid. A separate central line may be needed just for dialysis.

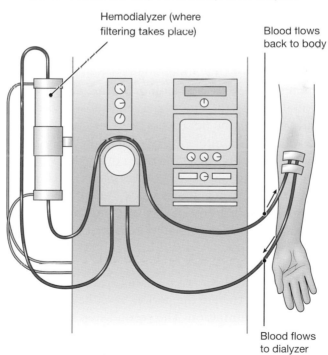

Hemodialyzer (where filtering takes place)

Blood flows back to body

Blood flows to dialyzer

Figure 8.2   Examples of Continuous Renal Replacement Therapy Machines

Continuous renal replacement therapy is a type of dialysis for patients with low blood pressure. The machine cleans the blood and removes fluid throughout the day and night.

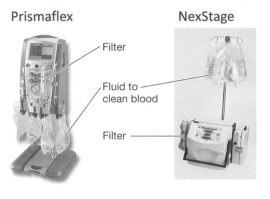

Prismaflex   NexStage

Filter

Fluid to
clean blood

Filter

Breathing

Basics About Breathing

Breathing is important for 2 reasons. First, patients need to breathe in (inhale) oxygen for their organs to work. Second, they need to breathe out (exhale) the "exhaust" of organs, carbon dioxide. If patients cannot breathe out enough carbon dioxide, they can become confused, sleepy, and stop breathing altogether. For a body to function normally, the lungs have to be able to breathe in oxygen (oxygenate) and breathe out carbon dioxide (ventilate).

The ICU team monitors the oxygen in the body continuously. This is done with a tool called the pulse oximeter, which is usually wrapped around the patient's finger and glows red. It reads the amount of oxygen in the patient's blood, called the oxygen saturation (sats). If this level falls below 92%, the ICU team may provide oxygen to the patient. The only way to see the patient's carbon dioxide level is to take a blood sample. The test is called an arterial blood gas, and it is described in Lab Tests (page 65).

When a patient is having trouble breathing, 2 actions are needed. The first is to help the patient breathe by providing oxygen and, if necessary, ventilation. The second step is to find out why the patient is having trouble breathing and fix that problem. There are many reasons for a patient's troubled breathing, and the ICU team will make those clear to the patient and family. The following sections explain the ways the ICU team helps the patient breathe.

Nurse's Note

■ If a patient's oxygen levels are decreasing, this is referred to as desatting.

■ It is OK for some patients to have oxygen saturation levels that are lower than 92%. If concerned, you can always ask your nurse what is appropriate for your loved one.

First Steps to Improve Breathing

If a patient is struggling to breathe, fixing their positioning in bed can help. It is harder to breathe when lying flat or slouching in bed. Therefore, a quick way to improve their oxygen level is to raise them up into a sitting position. Pain and anxiety can also make it difficult to breathe effectively. The staff tries to reduce both of these without medication. However, if the patient's oxygen level is too low, medication may be necessary to allow the patient to take full breaths.

Nurse's Note

■ If pain and anxiety are an issue, please see the sections, Managing Pain Without Medicine (page 51) and Mild Sedation (page 56) for tips to help your loved one breathe.

If the patient only needs a little help from oxygen, the ICU staff may use a <u>nasal cannula</u>. This thin tubing rests below the patient's nose, and it provides a small amount of oxygen (1-6 liters per minute [LPM]). How much oxygen is provided depends on the amount needed to keep the patient's oxygen levels greater than 92%.

As the amount of oxygen provided increases, the patient's nose and throat can dry out. An adapter may be available to add moisture to the air flowing through the nasal cannula. Additionally, if the tubing causes skin redness or hurts the ears, the nurse can provide ear protectors to prevent skin breakdown.

Nurse's Note

■ If your loved one prefers to breathe through the mouth, the nasal cannula is not as effective. Try to focus on breathing through the nose, especially if you notice the oxygen levels dropping.

■ Ask the nurse for a humidifier if the patient's nose is getting dry.

■ An incentive spirometer can also help increase oxygen levels. Ask the nurse if this is appropriate and how to use it.

Figure 8.3 Nasal Cannula

A nasal cannula is usually the first step when treating low oxygen levels. A humidifier and ear protectors improve comfort.

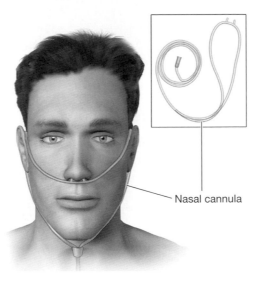

Nasal cannula

A Non-Rebreather Mask: Quick Increase in Oxygen Levels

The <u>non-rebreather</u> is a mask, connected to an oxygen-filled bag beneath, that covers the mouth and nose. It is called a non-rebreather because when the patient breathes out, the carbon dioxide flows outside of the mask. The mask then fills with oxygen from the connected bag. About 15 LPM of oxygen flow into the mask.

The non-rebreather is commonly worn by patients coming from the operating room and those who have a sudden need for more oxygen. It is easy to quickly set up, but it is not the best way to provide a large amount of oxygen. Because of this, it usually is temporary until a more efficient oxygen therapy is assembled.

Nurse's Note

- A venturi mask may be recommended for your loved one if they need more help than a nasal cannula. This is a mask that can give about 25% to 60% oxygen and can be worn for longer than a non-rebreather.

Figure 8.4 Non-Rebreather Mask

A non-rebreather is usually a short-term way to increase the patient's oxygen levels.

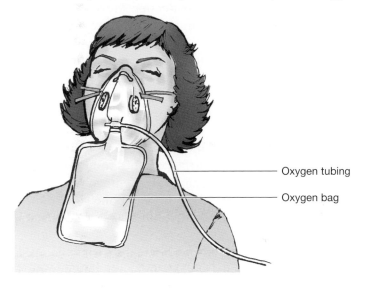

Oxygen tubing

Oxygen bag

Continuous Positive Airway Pressure and Bilevel Positive Airway Pressure: Aid for Sleep Apnea or High-Level Help for Breathing Difficulty

If lesser oxygen therapies are not providing enough support, the ICU staff can use a therapy that helps many adults, continuous positive airway pressure (CPAP). The CPAP machine is connected to a mask that covers the nose, the nose and mouth, or the entire face. It is usually worn to help prevent damage from sleep apnea, a serious condition where patients stop breathing for long periods during sleep. This causes small airways in the lungs to collapse, resulting in low oxygen levels. The CPAP continuously pushes air into the lungs, which helps to prevent those small airways from collapsing. The machine can also provide a higher percentage of oxygen for patients who have breathing difficulty combined with sleep apnea.

More help can be provided by bilevel positive airway pressure (BiPAP). While CPAP provides constant pressure, BiPAP pushes air into the lungs at 2 different levels. BiPAP machines can sense breathing in and out. On a breath in, it pushes at a higher pressure, and on a breath out, it lowers the pressure. This helps to keep the small airways in the lungs open and is more comfortable than CPAP. BiPAP can also provide a higher percentage of oxygen if needed.

BiPAP also serves a valuable second purpose: it helps the patient to breathe out more carbon dioxide. The higher pressure makes the patient breathe deeper. More carbon dioxide can then be exhaled. So BiPAP can help the patient breathe in more oxygen and breathe out more carbon dioxide. Because of these abilities, it can assist patients with serious difficulty breathing. However, if more help is needed, inserting a breathing tube is the next step.

CPAP and BiPAP machines are typically used while the patient is sleeping, but they can be worn all day if needed. Unfortunately, they can be uncomfortable to wear for long periods. The pressurized air dries out the patient's mouth, and having the mask strapped to their head can become uncomfortable. The mask is also annoying because talking through one is hard, it must be removed to eat or drink, and small air leaks can develop around it that set off alarms.

Worryingly, the patient may mistakenly take the mask off because of these problems, which can be life threatening. Oxygen levels drop quickly, and patients can die. Those with significant breathing problems need to keep the mask on and alert the medical staff if a break is needed. The respiratory therapist (RT) and nurse will continually adjust this setup to make sure it is working for the patient.

Nurse's Note

- Alert the nurse or RT before taking the mask off!
- Be careful when eating or drinking in between this therapy. If food or drink remains in the patient's mouth, the pressure from these machines can force it into their lungs. This aspiration can cause a serious lung infection.
- Lip balm can prevent the mouth from drying out.
- If uncomfortable, there may be other breathing settings or mask models that you can try. Ask the RT if any other options are available.
- If you are having trouble sleeping, sleep aids, such as melatonin and ear plugs may help.
- If you want to say something, it may be easier to communicate through phone texting or writing on a whiteboard. Ask the nurse if one is available.
- Ask the nurse or RT for padding for the face if you are wearing the mask for a long time. This will protect your skin.

Figure 8.5 Mask Types for Continuous Positive Airway Pressure (CPAP) and Bilevel Positive Airway Pressure (BiPAP)

CPAP and BiPAP are used to help with sleep apnea and severe breathing problems. The therapy may be more comfortable with a different size or type of mask.

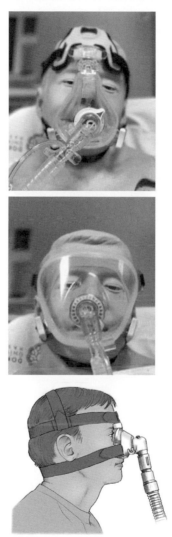

High-Flow Nasal Cannula: High-Level Help for Breathing Difficulty

A high-flow nasal cannula (HFNC), also called heated and humidified high-flow therapy, is a thin tube that delivers a precise percentage and flow of oxygen into the nose. The percentage can range from 21%, the amount of oxygen in regular air, to 100%, while flow rates can be set from 5 to 70 LPM. It can also help to remove carbon dioxide, but not as much as the BiPAP. However, it is more comfortable for prolonged use. The HFNC can be used to help patients with serious breathing difficulty. If this therapy does not provide enough oxygen, a breathing tube may be needed.

Worryingly, there is no alarm for the HFNC, and patients sometimes mistakenly remove it. This can be life threatening, and patients may die as a result. If a break is needed for any reason, the patient or family should alert the nurse or respiratory therapist (RT) to avoid a dangerous situation.

Nurse's Note

- Alert the nurse or RT before taking the HFNC off!
- Try to focus on breathing through the nose, especially if you notice the oxygen levels are dropping.
- Ask the nurse if it is OK to eat and drink. The high flow increases the risk of choking, and the flow level may have to be lowered while eating to make it safe.

Figure 8.6   High-Flow Nasal Cannula

The high-flow nasal cannula helps with severe breathing problems.

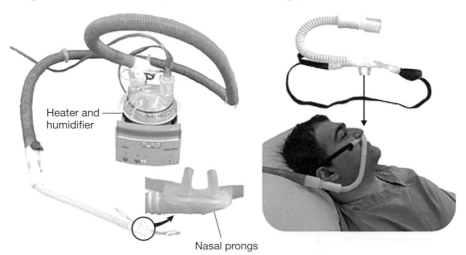

Heater and humidifier

Nasal prongs

The Ventilator: Total Help Breathing

The breathing machine, or <u>ventilator</u>, is common in every ICU. The ventilator, or vent, is programmed to deliver breaths that are customized for the patient. There are many different settings, but the main starting point is whether the ventilator begins a breath for the patient or assists a breath the patient started. Other options the medical team can adjust are the breathing rate, percentage of oxygen, and the amount of pressure and volume to fill the lungs.

The breathing tube, or <u>endotracheal tube</u>, connects the patient to the ventilator. It is inserted into the windpipe, or trachea, through the mouth. There is an inflatable ring, or cuff, at the bottom that stabilizes the tube in position. The tube is secured to a sticker placed on the patient's cheeks.

Nurse's Note

- Families commonly view the breathing tube and ventilator as life support. Although true, many other therapies in the ICU also count as life support. For instance, medication to raise blood pressure and machines to help the body function are included in this category.

- When you or your loved one does not want a breathing tube, it is called <u>do not intubate</u> (DNI). In this case, the breathing therapies mentioned earlier are used to help the patient breathe. Please see the Goals of Care section for further guidance on this topic (page 135).

Figure 8.7 The Ventilator (Breathing Machine)

The ventilator provides the most breathing support possible to the patient. Pictured are three examples of ventilators. Each has a control screen and tubing that connects to the patient.

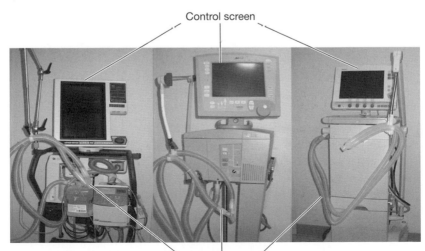

Control screen

Ventilator tubing

Respiratory Distress and Respiratory Failure: When Trouble Breathing Turns Into Needing a Breathing Tube

A patient who is having trouble breathing is experiencing what is called <u>respiratory distress</u>. Signs of this include feeling anxious or short of breath, breathing rapidly (more than 20 times per minute), being unable to speak in full sentences, or using abdominal and neck muscles to help breathe. These signs show that a patient is trying to reverse the low oxygen or high carbon dioxide levels in their body.

Respiratory distress turns into <u>respiratory failure</u> when the patient cannot breathe in enough oxygen. Respiratory failure also occurs if a patient cannot breathe out enough air, causing carbon dioxide to build up. For example, patients can only breathe quickly for so long before they get tired. When this happens, they breathe in less oxygen and breathe out less carbon dioxide, making them worse. Eventually, they stop breathing.

If the patient stops breathing, the brain, heart, and other organs are damaged from the lack of oxygen. This damage can happen quickly. So, it is important to avoid any interruption in the patient's breathing. Therefore, if a patient in respiratory distress looks to be tiring, the medical team discusses inserting the breathing tube. This is known as <u>intubation</u>. Although it can be upsetting to family, intubation means the patient is safer. It gives the ICU team better control of a dangerous situation.

Nurse's Note

- The medical team may decide to intubate before respiratory failure. This avoids an emergency and any damage from respiratory failure.
- The medical team may intubate patients who cannot be woken up. These patients may stop breathing and suffer injury from the lack of oxygen. A breathing tube will make sure they can receive oxygen.

Intubation: Inserting the Breathing Tube

The breathing tube is inserted with a procedure known as <u>intubation</u>. First, 100% oxygen is given to the patient. This is done with a bag valve mask, or Ambu bag. This mask is held to the patient's face, and the connected bag of oxygen is squeezed. This helps patients who are struggling to breathe by pushing oxygen into their lungs. The ICU staff then gives a sedative followed by a temporary paralytic. These medications make the patient comfortable and minimize their movement so the breathing tube can be rapidly inserted. Once in place, it is attached to the ventilator.

The correct location of the breathing tube is confirmed with an X-ray. Given the need to act quickly, the family typically is asked to wait outside during the procedure.

It is stressful being at the bedside of a loved one with a breathing tube. Families should be assured that the nurse and medical team are continuously monitoring these patients to make sure they are safe and comfortable.

Figure 8.8   Bag Valve Mask

A bag valve mask is used to help increase the patient's oxygen levels before inserting the breathing tube.

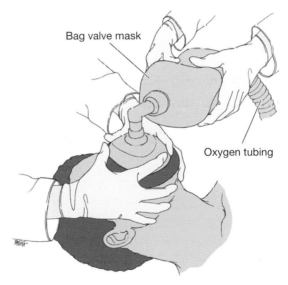

Figure 8.9 Endotracheal Tube (Breathing Tube)

The endotracheal tube is inserted into the trachea and secured in place with an inflatable cuff. A tube holder or tape secures it to the face, and it is connected to the ventilator tubing.

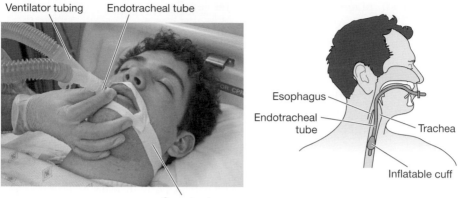

Securing tape

9

Essentials for the ICU Patient

Many different types of intensive care unit (ICU) patients need similar therapies to recover and prevent complications. These therapies are remembered by the letters in FASTHUGS BID—*Feeding, Analgesic, Sedation, Thromboembolic prevention, Head of bed elevated, Ulcer prevention, Glucose control, Spontaneous breathing trial, Bowel regimen, Indwelling catheter removal*, and *De-escalation of antibiotics*. Some hospitals may have a different name than FASTHUGS BID, but all ICUs use these therapies. Because they are important for patient recovery, each of these topics is reviewed in rounds every morning.

This section outlines FASTHUGS BID and 4 other critical parts of recovery, the "get to know me" board, the ICU journal, removing the breathing tube, and early mobility.

These therapies are important to consider for all ICU patients. However, some of them do not apply to certain patients and will therefore not be used. For instance, if a breathing tube is not needed, the related therapies will not occur. Additionally, some of these topics are discussed in more detail elsewhere. For more information on the topics, please see the included page numbers. As always, the medical team can answer any questions the patient or family has.

Figure 9.1 Equipment in the ICU Room

This picture shows some of the therapies used to treat patients. In the ICU there may be more or less equipment present depending on the illness.

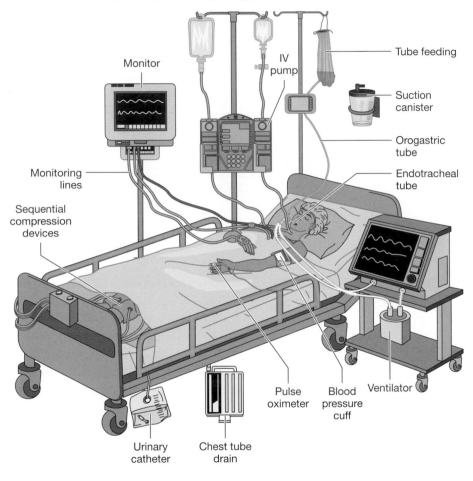

Feeding: Providing Nutrition to Help Recovery

Food helps patients recover. Feeding begins as soon as possible, as long as it can happen safely. It can be delayed for some procedures or illnesses.

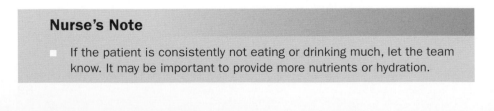

Nurse's Note

■ If the patient is consistently not eating or drinking much, let the team know. It may be important to provide more nutrients or hydration.

A patient with a breathing tube also receives nutrition. Generally, feeding begins if the breathing tube will be needed for longer than 2 days. When the breathing tube is inserted, another smaller tube is placed alongside it that ends in the stomach. This smaller tube can enter through the mouth (orogastric, OG) or nose (nasogastric, NG). Through this tube, the patient is given liquid nutrition, or tube feeds. It usually runs continuously, and water will flush the tube every so often to provide hydration. The dietician customizes the amount of nutrition given depending on the patient's needs. Patients also receive medicine through this tube.

The OG and NG can increase the risk of a lung infection. This can happen when fluid travels from the stomach, up the esophagus, and into the back of the throat. From there, it can leak down into the lungs. This is called aspiration. When anything that is not supposed to be in the lungs gets in there, aspiration occurs. Scarily, it can happen without any signs, such as choking or coughing, and it can cause a dangerous infection. To prevent this, nurses monitor for a buildup of fluid in the stomach, suction out fluid from the mouth, and keep the head of the bed elevated as often as possible.

If the medical team is especially worried about aspiration, a nasoduodenal tube (ND) may be chosen. It can reduce the risk of aspiration because it is inserted through the nose, passes through the stomach, and ends just past the stomach in the small intestine. This prevents fluids from traveling up the esophagus, and therefore reduces the possibility for aspiration. Another benefit of a ND is that there is less risk of skin breakdown compared to the NG and OG, so it can be used for longer.

If the patient will need tube feeds for more than a few weeks, another type of feeding tube is considered. The percutaneous endoscopic gastrostomy (PEG) tube is placed through the abdomen into the stomach. Another option is a jejunostomy (J) tube, which is inserted just past the stomach in the small intestine. Both options can be combined in one tube, and this is called a G/J tube. Tube feeds are given through the J tube to prevent the risk of aspiration, while the stomach access is for medication.

Patients who cannot absorb nutrients through their stomach or intestines can receive nutrition through an IV directly into their blood. This is known as total parenteral nutrition (TPN). It provides a complex mixture of nutrients that runs continuously into the patient.

See Figure 4.7 (page 36) for the different types of feeding tubes.

Analgesic: Reducing Pain

Patients can experience pain from both medical devices and their illness. Recovering from an operation, battling a lung infection, or simply having a breathing tube can be painful. Unfortunately, pain can slow a patient's recovery or even reverse progress already made.

Managing pain is important for every patient, including those with a breathing tube. The ICU staff uses medicinal and nonmedicinal tools to manage pain. The medical team can change the strategy based on pain ratings or, if the patient cannot talk, signs of discomfort. For instance, pain may cause an increase in breathing rate, heart rate, blood pressure, facial grimacing, or tense muscles. Nurses are required to assess pain levels often. Please see the sections on pain in Chapter 5, page 49, for more information.

Sedation: Relaxation During Extended Therapy

Many illnesses and procedures can cause discomfort and anxiety. Sedation medication can reduce these symptoms. Importantly, they also help the patient relax enough to allow the medical care to work. For example, when not sedated, a patient may instinctively try to breathe against the air provided by the ventilator. This prevents the therapy from helping the patient recover. Sedation allows the patient to relax and lets the ventilator work for them.

Most ventilated patients continuously receive sedation medication. Ideally, the patient is comfortable while still being sleepily responsive to the caregiver.

The sedation is paused daily for most patients. This is called a sedation vacation or a spontaneous awakening trial. During this time when the patient is more awake, the ICU team tests the patient to make sure no brain injuries have occurred. Brain injuries are not caused by sedation, but they are harder to detect when the patient is less responsive. The sedation vacation is also an opportunity to reduce the amount of sedation needed. The goal is to use the least amount of medication possible for the medical care to work for the patient. If the patient shows signs of distress that may hurt their recovery, the sedation may be resumed. Please see Deep Sedation, page 57, for more information.

Nurse's Note

- A sedation vacation may not occur if a patient's therapy depends on uninterrupted sedation.

- Some patients say they hear and remember things during sedation. Most patients say they cannot remember anything that happened while sedated. Holding the patient's hand and speaking to them can be soothing for the patient and family. Check with the nurse first to make sure this is OK.

Thromboembolic Prevention: Preventing Blood Clots

When people are less active, like many ICU patients, their blood flow slows down. This increases the risk of blood cells sticking together and forming a blood clot, called a thrombus. When this occurs in a vein, it is called a deep vein thrombosis (DVT). This blood clot becomes more dangerous if it gets caught in a blood vessel and blocks blood flow. When this occurs, the blood clot is then called an embolus. When blood flow is cut off, tissue downstream from the blockage dies. This can be life threatening if it occurs in the lungs or brain.

To help prevent blood clots, patients are given medications known as blood thinners, or anticoagulants. Heparin and enoxaparin are examples of blood thinners. Usually, they are given by injection into the patient's belly fat. Also, shin massagers or stockings are used to help squeeze the blood back toward the heart, preventing it from slowing and clotting in the legs. The massagers are called sequential compression devices (SCDs), and the stockings are called thromboembolic deterrent (TED) hose.

Importantly, getting out of bed, or mobilizing, is critical to prevent blood clots. This should occur as soon as possible, and some hospitals do this before the breathing tube is removed. Even patients who cannot get out of bed can exercise with physical therapy (OT) and occupational therapy (OT) to increase blood flow.

Nurse's Note

■ Some blood thinners need to be stopped before procedures to prevent bleeding. If an invasive procedure is scheduled, ask the medical team if the blood thinner needs to be stopped a certain amount of time before.

Figure 9.2   The Danger of Blood Clots

A blood clot that blocks blood flow in a vein is called a deep vein thrombosis (DVT). It typically affects only one leg, which can become more swollen, painful, redder, or warmer than the other. A DVT can detach and become lodged downstream, blocking blood flow in the lungs or brain. This is called an embolus (see Figure 9.3, page x). The ICU team tries to prevent this with medicine, movement, and tools to promote blood flow.

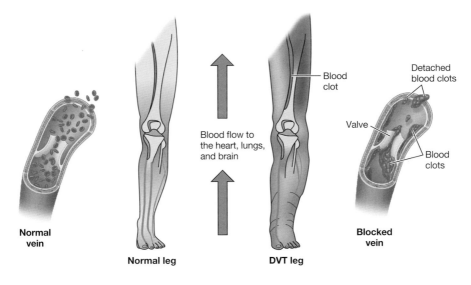

Normal vein

Normal leg

Blood flow to the heart, lungs, and brain

Blood clot

DVT leg

Detached blood clots

Valve

Blood clots

Blocked vein

Figure 9.3 Brain Injury From a Blood Clot

Blood clots travel throughout the body in the blood. When a blood clot blocks the blood flow in the brain, it is called a cerebral embolism. This blockage starves downstream tissue of oxygen, injuring the brain. The resulting brain injury is called an ischemic stroke.

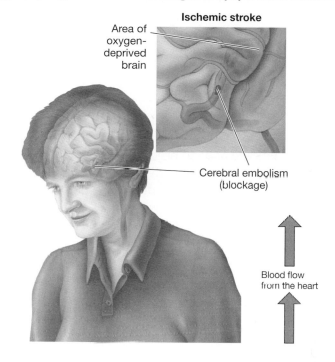

Ischemic stroke

Area of oxygen-deprived brain

Cerebral embolism (blockage)

Blood flow from the heart

Head of Bed Elevation: Preventing Lung Infections

Lung infections, or pneumonia, can occur in the ICU. One way is when food or liquid gets into the patient's lungs, called aspiration. The risk of aspiration can be reduced by making sure the patient is fully awake, sitting upright, and has been cleared by the nurse to eat or drink. Patients who have trouble eating or drinking have to pass a swallow test (page 41).

Pneumonia can be life threatening for ICU patients. ICU patients, especially if it occurs in patients with a breathing tube. This is a condition called ventilator-associated pneumonia (VAP).

One way to prevent VAP is to sit patients up by elevating the head of their bed (about 30°). This prevents stomach contents from traveling up the esophagus where they can be aspirated. This also prevents saliva and stomach contents from pooling in the back of the mouth. There, pneumonia-causing bacteria can grow and get into the lungs. Finally, this position gives the ICU staff a better angle to suction out the harmful fluid.

The medical team is always watching for signs of pneumonia, such as fever, increased white blood cell count, a new cough, or an increase or discoloration of sputum (phlegm). Both the breathing tube and the patient's mouth are suctioned routinely to prevent a buildup of fluid. However, the patient may not be suctioned frequently in order to prevent throat irritation or bleeding. If pneumonia is suspected, a culture of the sputum is taken, and the patient is started on antibiotics.

Ulcer Prevention: Preventing Stomach Damage

Any illness causes the body to produce stress chemicals. They can cause damage throughout the body. The ICU staff tries to reduce the amount of these chemicals by decreasing stress (using sedation, reducing pain, encouraging exercise, etc).

One way the body reacts to stress chemicals is by producing more stomach acid. This can destroy the protective lining of the stomach and lead to a sore, or ulcer. Stomach pain and bleeding can occur as a result.

To prevent an ulcer from developing, medicine is given to limit the overproduction of stomach acid. Examples of this medicine are pantoprazole, famotidine, and sucralfate.

Glucose Control: Managing Blood Sugar

Blood sugar, or glucose, is the main source of energy in the body. It is important to have the right amount of blood sugar because both too little and too much can hurt the patient. Too little blood sugar can cause the body to shut down because it does not have the energy to function. However, high levels of sugar in the blood can act as food for bacteria. This increases the risk for infection. Wounds also do not heal well when blood sugar levels are high.

Stress chemicals, which every patient makes, reduce the body's ability to use glucose. So, more sugar remains in the blood. Additionally, nutrition and some medications, such as steroids, can also increase blood sugar levels.

Patients recover best when their blood sugar levels are kept between 140 and 180. Because this is important, blood sugar levels are checked regularly, sometimes as often as every hour. Additionally, insulin may be prescribed to keep those levels in check. This medication helps the body use blood sugar. Many patients need insulin in the hospital, even if they do not take it at home or have diabetes. The provider can advise if insulin will be needed after the hospital.

Spontaneous Breathing Trial: Testing if the Breathing Tube Can Be Removed

Before the breathing tube is taken out, the patient must be able to safely breathe on their own. To test if a patient can support their own breathing, the ICU team reduces the amount of help supplied by the ventilator. This test is called a spontaneous breathing trial (SBT), and it occurs after reducing the amount of sedation medication. The SBT usually happens when the patient needs only about 30% oxygen.

Some providers decide to remove the breathing tube based on a lab called an arterial blood gas. This shows the balance of oxygen and carbon dioxide in the blood caused by the patient's breathing. Following a failed SBT, this test would show low oxygen levels and high carbon dioxide levels. Other medical teams measure lung strength to see if they are too weak to breathe unassisted. Some ICUs watch patients to see if they are breathing too fast, dropping their oxygen levels, not following commands, or looking distressed. If these occur, the patient may not be ready to have the breathing tube removed. However, if these issues are not present, the breathing tube may be ready to come out. Please see the section on removing the breathing tube, Extubation, page 100.

Bowel Regimen: Promoting Bowel Movements

Many patients experience constipation while in the hospital. Usually, they are not walking as much, eating enough fiber, or drinking enough fluids—all of which contribute to fewer bowel movements. Opioid pain medications also cause constipation.

If this issue is not treated, discomfort, nausea, and vomiting occur. If constipation continues, the patient cannot eat, which slows recovery. Furthermore, bowel movements are necessary for ridding the body of toxic substances and keeping electrolytes balanced. Therefore, it is important to keep a regular schedule.

Medications to avoid constipation can be prescribed. These can include stool softeners, stool bulkers, and laxatives to help move the bowels. If needed, more immediately effective tools can be used, such as suppositories or enemas. Exercising also helps to prevent constipation.

Indwelling Catheter Removal: Preventing Infection of Lines

An ICU patient may need many catheters for their treatment. Examples of these include peripheral IVs, chest tubes, central lines, and urinary catheters. Once no longer needed, they should be removed to reduce the risk of infection. It is especially important to see if central lines or the urinary catheter can be removed. An infection from these lines can be life threatening. So, the ICU team assesses if they can be removed each day.

De-escalation of Antibiotics: Targeting the Infection

If an infection is suspected, the patient is started on antibiotics that kill many types of germs (broad spectrum). A sample of fluid, called a culture, taken from the infected area, identifies the type of germ and which antibiotic can kill that germ. The patient is then switched to the antibiotic that targets the known germ (narrow spectrum). Reducing the number of antibiotics given to the patient by precisely targeting the infection is called de-escalation. This reduces side effects of the antibiotics and prevents the development of antibiotic-resistant germs.

The "Get to Know Me" Board: Helping Everyone Know the Patient

Patients on the ventilator, as well as some other ICU patients, are not as responsive as they usually are. Additionally, the patient in the bed may have a different personality now, compared to before they became ill. Also, family members may feel unfamiliar with the patient who now looks or acts differently than in their usual life. These changes can be upsetting in an already distressing environment. What can be comforting is to connect the patient in the room to who they are outside of the hospital. Additionally, knowing more about the patient's personality helps the medical team when caring for their mind and body.

The "get to know me" board makes these ideas happen. Placed in the room, the family lists the patient's preferred name, favorite

activities, proud accomplishments, what makes him or her ner-
vous, and a few other tidbits. There are also spaces for pictures.
Celebrating the patient's personality can ease anxiety, and the staff
enjoy learning more about the patient.

Nurse's Note

■ If there is no board available, ask the nurse if you can make one and
put it up in the room. Please see Appendix 3 for some ideas (page
184). Feel free to add anything you think is important to know.

ICU Journal: Better Insight for Now and Later

The patient and family have many experiences over the course of
an ICU stay. Because many things happen quickly, it can be hard
to remember and process everything at once. Writing about these
events and detailing the thoughts in these moments can be helpful.
By describing the situation, what was said, and feelings during those
times, patients and families can create a guide to revisit later for a
better understanding.

Often, patients do not remember some of their time in the
ICU. A journal, written by family, can help them grasp what happened and provide meaning to those times that may have been life
changing. Furthermore, many patients and families suffer from
post-intensive care syndrome after leaving the ICU (see How to
Prepare Now for a Better Life After Hospitalization, page 105). By
keeping a journal, the patient and family can help themselves avoid
this issue.

Nurse's Note

■ Feel free to ask the staff to write in your journal about the day, any
change, important events, etc.
■ Please see Appendix 2 for a journal outline (page 177).

Extubation: Removing the Breathing Tube

After a patient passes the spontaneous breathing trial (SBT), the breathing tube is removed. This is called extubation.

Removing the breathing tube is quick and painless. Usually, family can stay in the room if they like. The respiratory therapist (RT) removes the tape securing the tube and deflates the cuff in the trachea. Instructing the patient to cough and to not swallow, the RT pulls the tube out while suctioning any fluids in the mouth. Oxygen is given if the patient needs it.

After removing the breathing tube, the patient may have a sore throat and hoarse voice for a couple of days. They can use a numbing throat spray or suck on ice chips to reduce this pain. Before the patient can eat or drink, they need to pass a swallow test (page 41). Another important piece to the patient's recovery is to make their lungs stronger. This is done with an incentive spirometer, which the nurse teaches the patient how to use.

Nurse's Note

- After removing the breathing tube, ask the nurse if it is OK for the patient to eat or drink anything.
- The family is a great resource for encouraging and reminding the patient to use the incentive spirometer. Go for a record!

Early Mobility: Exercising ASAP

Staying in bed called bedrest, negatively affects every part of the body. Getting patients out of bed, or mobilizing, as soon as possible helps them recover faster. This provides countless benefits, such as reducing the risk of pressure injuries and blood clots, lessening the need for stool softeners, stimulating appetite, improving sleep quality, gaining strength, and exercising the muscles, heart, and lungs. It is also another accomplishment to celebrate with the patient.

The staff tries to encourage mobility in any safe way possible. This can range from sitting at the edge of the bed to walking. Often, patients need to be persuaded to get out of bed because they feel fatigued, weak, in pain, or even hopeless. However, nearly all patients say they are happy they exercised afterward. The experts on movement are the the physical therapists (PTs), occupational therapists (OTs), and mobility technicians. They know the best ways to motivate and mobilize patients safely. They usually visit several times per week.

Nurse's Note

- Preparing for PT or OT is important for a good session. If pain is an issue, request pain medicine before the workout. A coffee or nap before therapy can also help get your loved one ready. You can also ask to schedule the workout during a time that is best for the patient.
- Encourage patients when they are working with PT and OT. Celebrate their accomplishment afterward with them. It is hard, but important, work.
- Ask the PT or OT for homework—exercises that can be done when the PT and OT are not there. This extra effort makes patients readier to go home!
- Even if PT or OT are not scheduled, you can ask the nurse to sit in a chair or go for a walk.

10

How to Help the Patient During Downtime

Patients and families often find the intensive care unit (ICU) challenging in many ways. Being at a loved one's bedside, even for short periods of time, can be exhausting physically and emotionally. The noisy machines, the confusion of days turning to nights and back, and inconsistent sleep are just a few of the challenges in an already stressful environment. Complicating these difficult times are the surprising and unexpected setbacks that may follow joyful patient improvements. Often, the future remains uncertain.

In many cases, patients cannot interact with family as they normally do because of exhaustion, delirium, or the medical therapy. In these times, even the most resilient family can feel helpless and isolated as they wait for results. This is especially difficult for family members who are used to providing for their loved one's basic needs. Now that they cannot care for the patient, they feel a sense of emptiness or loss of purpose. Alternatively, others may have been disconnected with their now-sick relative. Being unable to make up for the lost time can be upsetting. They may feel a sense of needing to provide extra care now, even if it is not needed. And, of course, many family members simply want to help in any way they can.

Luckily, there are ways to make a positive impact for those loved ones in the ICU. Although it can feel scary, the family is welcome to provide some patient care. In addition to making the patient look and feel better, many families say these acts help to reduce anxiety during the hospital stay and after the patient leaves.

A great way to start is by asking what help the nurse can use. Even small acts, such as helping the patient to brush their teeth, folding the unused linen, assisting the patient to a drink, or organizing the patient's things within arm's reach, can help a busy nurse focus more on medical care.

Another option is to help the patient with the exercises left by the physical therapist, occupational therapist, speech-language pathologist, and nurse. Families can encourage and remind the patient that these are important. They can also ask for extra exercises to further improve their recovery.

Often a patient's appearance is different than usual because their hygiene is hospital focused (eg, giving patients baths to prevent infection). One of the most comforting acts can be a sponge bath with warm water and washcloths. Patients can be given a shampoo or shave, if time and medical care allow. Even using a damp towel to clean the face or applying lip balm can go a long way. Also, brushing or braiding hair can be soothing and helps restore the patient's pre-hospital appearance. Moisturizing cream can be applied to prevent dry and damaged skin. Using the moisturizer to massage the muscles increases blood flow and comforts the patient. The nurse can provide these grooming tools and mention any important tips.

Another valuable opportunity to aid in recovery is to create a stimulating and familiar environment to help motivate patients, comfort them, and prevent confusion. Bringing in family pictures, playing familiar and relaxing music, and talking or reading to patients help these goals. Some patients who cannot respond or are sedated, later say they could hear during that time. So, interaction may still be comforting for those patients.

However, it is important not to overdo the stimulation because patients need to rest in order to recover. Family members can also, with good intentions, coddle patients. Patients need to help themselves get better by doing things for themselves. Therefore, if they can feed themselves, let them do it. If they can fix their own blanket, let them reach down and accomplish this. Encouraging this is not being mean. It is part of the ICU team and family effort to empower patients for when they get out of the hospital. Any gaps will be filled in when help is needed. The ICU team can answer any questions or concerns the family has about this.

It is also equally important that the family learn to take care of themselves. Patients will not be in the ICU forever. When the patient goes home, the family may then be providing most of the care. In order to prepare for those moments to come, it is critical that the family takes time off during the long nights and stressful days.

Therefore, while in the ICU, let the medical team take care of the patient. The staff keeps an eye on the patient for 24 hours each day of the week. Family members should go for a walk and get some fresh air. Get something to eat besides hospital food. Go home or back to the hotel and take a shower. Or better yet, a relaxing bath. Rest and get some sleep. Let another family member take a shift at the bedside. Let the nurse care for the patient, as they do every day. The nurse will call if anything changes. As nurses often say, "We will be here all night."

11

How to Prepare Now for a Better Life After Hospitalization
Post-Intensive Care Syndrome

The intensive care unit (ICU) experience is difficult for those in the bed and those next to it. Surviving the illness and leaving the hospital is a major accomplishment. However, this is not when healing stops. Unfortunately, a stay in the ICU can stick with patients and with families, even those who did not lose a loved one.

After leaving the hospital, many patients and families have problems with their mind, body, and emotions. These problems are common. They are part of <u>post-intensive care syndrome</u> (PICS) and <u>post-intensive care syndrome–family</u> (PICS-F; to simplify, PICS-F is included in PICS, unless noted). Because of the stressors of the ICU, PICS can last for years after leaving the hospital. PICS affects the body, mind, and emotions in ways that make getting back to regular life harder.

Nurse's Note

- This next part can be upsetting. However, you have to be prepared for what could lay ahead, so this information had to be included. After learning about PICS you will be able to prevent or address it. Strategies to do this are included. By reading this book and being interested in getting better, you will be prepared.

- The odds are that you will be affected by PICS.

- There are ways to help prevent PICS while in the hospital. Try to do these as much as possible.

- Some of the ways PICS can affect your life are mentioned. However, PICS can change other parts of your life. The sooner you recognize these changes and mention them to your healthcare provider, the sooner you can recover.

For patients, a common problem with their bodies after a critical illness is muscle weakness from the time spent in bed. This makes getting out of bed or walking harder. These patients also tire out quickly and need more rest. As a result, it is harder to exercise, more likely a fall will occur, and tiring to do simple tasks like getting dressed or making dinner.

Patients and families with PICS probably will have trouble controlling their emotions. They may feel anxious or depressed even if they are not currently experiencing anything scary or sad. PICS may cause someone to be uninterested in doing things they once liked, be tired all of the time, or not be able to sleep. Another common problem is anxiety with things that are a reminder of the ICU. This causes patients and families to avoid those things, even if they are important. For example, a patient with PICS may not want to work with physical therapy because it reminds them of their time in the ICU. This makes it harder to get stronger. The name for this is post-traumatic stress disorder (PTSD), which can occur with PICS. PTSD may also cause patients to worry too much about things that might happen, such as getting sick again. Nightmares or reliving experiences from the ICU may occur as well. Each of these problems with emotions can hurt relationships, prevent those affected from getting help, and limit the ability to enjoy life.

PICS can also cause patients and families to have trouble with their minds. Many people say they have problems concentrating, remembering details, planning events, or making decisions. Thinking can take more effort or time to complete. Also, people with PICS may struggle to say exactly what they are thinking. These issues can make it difficult to return to work, hang out with friends, cook dinner, or plan a trip.

In some ways, troubles with the mind and emotions are more frustrating than problems with the body. A physical problem can be seen, while injuries to the mind and emotions are hidden. So, some people wrongly assume that if the body is healthy, then the mind and emotions should be fine. Also, some people think the patient should feel happy because they are well enough to leave the hospital. Unfortunately, those with PICS may also share these thoughts. Each patient is different and recovers at their own speed. Just as some patients need specific medicine to recover, PICS can be helped with specific medical care. Importantly, without help, these issues may get worse. Recognizing and communicating these problems to a health professional is the best step toward getting better.

Nurse's Note

- You are not alone. Many people experience the symptoms of PICS.
- The odds are that you will have PICS, and without help it will not get better.
- How much help you need should not be the focus. What is important is that there is room to get better, and any step toward that recovery will benefit you.

Worryingly, PICS can make it harder to recover outside of the hospital. For instance, patients may have to meet with providers to discuss their recovery. Getting to this follow-up appointment requires making a plan, remembering and following the plan, being strong enough to get to the appointment, and not avoiding or becoming overwhelmed by the continued medical attention. All of these steps need to happen to get better, and PICS can get in the way of each one.

For family, PICS-F can hurt the ability to return to everyday life in big and small ways. The stress or trouble sleeping may make family feel anxious or on-edge with everything their loved one does. These issues can be made worse by financial problems, such as lost work and medical bills. And, if a loved one dies in the ICU, those with PICS-F may have feelings of sadness, anxiety, guilt, betrayal, or resentment for many months after the hospital stay. This is called complicated grief. Each of these issues can hurt the family member's ability to care for themselves and others.

Nurse's Note

■ Family may feel as if they should not need help recovering, or they may feel guilty for having these symptoms because they were not sick. However, the ICU can affect family as much as patients. Recognizing the signs of PICS-F and communicating them to a healthcare professional is important for getting better.

Preventing and Overcoming Post-Intensive Care Syndrome

There are ways to help prevent or overcome the effects of PICS. These tips are for patients and families during the hospital stay and after discharge. They may not all be available, but doing as many as possible will give the best chance for limiting PICS. As always, the medical team is available to answer any questions and give suggestions.

How the Patient and Family Can Limit PICS During and After the Hospitalization

■ Notice the signs of PICS and communicate them with the medical team, a primary care provider, or a mental health professional. This is the best step to getting help.
■ Be active during the day (exercise, work with physical and occupational therapy, take a walk, etc).
■ Try to sleep only during the night.
■ Prevent delirium (see Delirium, page 66).
■ Treat the body well (quit smoking, eat healthy, limit alcohol, etc).
■ Keep a journal of the experience (see ICU Journal, page 99, Appendix 2 for an outline, page 177).
■ Keep in contact with family and friends as much as possible. These social connections are important for support, remaining close to those who matter, and returning to regular life. They can also help you with responsibilities. A good way to start this is through online resources, such as CaringBridge (please visit NavigatingTheICU.com for the link).

- Online or in-person support groups are available to connect with those who know what the ICU experience and recovery are like and can share tips, stories, etc. They can be found through the social worker, spiritual services, healthcare plans, and groups (with links at NavigatingTheICU.com) such as the following:
  - HealthUnlocked
  - Inspire
  - Healthtalk, which offers stories from patients and families in the ICU
- Patients and families often struggle with how to include or not include children in an ICU stay. This is especially true with end-of-life care. Hospitals may have access to staff who specialize in helping children visit the ICU. The nurse knows how to reach them.
- PICS clinics specialize in taking care of patients and families with PICS once they are out of the hospital. They are only available in some areas. The social worker, case manager, or an online search may be able to find one close to you.

The most important step is recognizing any of the symptoms of PICS and telling a medical professional.

Nurse's Note

- Even if you do not need help, mentioning that you are feeling the effects of PICS to a healthcare professional is valuable. That way you both can be prepared if help is needed.
- Communication with others is important. Although family and friends may be frustrating or fussy, they are this way because they care about you. These relationships offer support and are important for getting better, so they must be treated with kindness.

Additional Ways the Patient Can Prevent PICS During the Hospitalization

- Talk to the nurse, provider, social worker, case manager, and spiritual services about ways to sleep better, relieve stress, reduce pain, and prevent PICS.
- Request to see a mental health professional if there are problems with the mind or emotions.

- Before leaving the hospital, have the medical team fill out a brief ICU stay form (accessed by visiting NavigatingTheICU.com). This should be given to the primary care provider. It mentions what happened during the ICU stay and alerts the provider to look out for signs of PICS.

Additional Ways the Patient Can Limit PICS After the Hospitalization

- Work out the muscles, lungs, and heart.
  - Physical and occupational therapy may need to continue outside of the hospital.
  - Those with heart and lung problems may benefit from working with experts in heart and lung recovery (cardiac and pulmonary rehabilitation).

Additional Ways the Family Can Prevent PICS-F During the Hospitalization

For families, supporting a loved one in the ICU is a marathon. The family has to prepare themselves for the long road ahead, especially since the patient may need support after leaving the hospital. It is harder to help the patient's body, mind, and emotions recover when the family is struggling with PICS-F. In addition to those tips mentioned earlier in this section, below are others that can help the family.

- Be present for rounds (see Chapter 2, page 8, and Appendix 1 for a rounding guide, page 163).
- Interact with the healthcare team (ask questions, mention important patient values, etc).
- Set up a time for patient updates with the nurse and/or provider.
- Visit the patient.
- Video call with the patient.
- Talk to the patient.[*]
- Help the patient exercise.[*]
- Help groom the patient.[*]
- Talk to the nurse, provider, social worker, case manager, and spiritual services about ways to prevent PICS and PICS-F.

    Other helpful ways to relieve stress include the following:

- Take a break from the ICU. A change of scenery for any amount of time can help relieve stress. Even a short walk to the cafeteria

---

[*]Check with the nurse to make sure this is OK for the patient's recovery.

for a coffee helps. Another option is to take shifts with other family members or friends. One family member stays at the bedside while the other takes a break, sleeps, exercises, runs errands, etc.

- Many hospitals can recommend nearby hotels that discount rooms for families of patients.
- Being unable to take care of responsibilities outside of the hospital can be upsetting. If friends and family ask how they can help, accept the assistance. They can bring in food, pick up the mail, take a pet for a walk, etc.
- Updating everyone each time something happens can be stressful. It is OK to set boundaries and limits so you can focus on what is important. You can say that you will update everyone at a certain time of the week, or you can ask one friend or family member to update everyone else. Also, using online resources to update everyone at once and asking for help can reduce the stress. One option is CaringBridge (link available at NavigatingTheICU.com).

Resource for the Family About How to Limit PICS-F After the Hospitalization

- The National Alliance for Caregiving website has information and advice for caregivers. It is a great resource to use in addition to the advice from medical professionals (link available at NavigatingTheICU.com).

12

Where the Patient Recovers After the Hospital

Patients may still need help recovering after leaving the hospital. This help can range from continued assistance from the ventilator to improving balance with physical therapy. Where this recovery occurs and for how long depends on how much help the patient needs. The medical team works together to make sure this decision is safe and follows the patient's goals of care (page 135).

Planning for recovery starts in the intensive care unit (ICU), and the family should begin this process as soon as possible. Although there may not be clear answers now, it is important to discuss the patient's recovery with the medical team and think about what the return home will look like. This gives the family the most time to prepare and head off any problems (see the end of this chapter for some questions).

Recovery after illness can be referred to as rehabilitation, or rehab. Its goal is to improve the patient's independence and help the patient return to their desired way of life. Rehab requires many days of hard work, which can make the journey challenging. This is especially true for those with post-intensive care syndrome (Chapter 11, page 105). With the help of the hospital's medical team, those providing care in rehab, and family, the patient can be given the best chance to recover.

The amount of help the patient needs determines their level of rehab. The types of rehab are mentioned below.

Long-Term Acute Care Hospital

Patients who still have significant medical needs, but do not need the life-saving interventions of the ICU, live in a long-term acute care hospital (LTACH). For example, patients who need help from the ventilator or have significant brain injury may benefit from this hospital-like setting.

Inpatient Rehabilitation Facility

Patients who can tolerate intense rehab (3 hours per day for 5 days per week) may live in an inpatient rehabilitation facility (IRF). These patients have medical needs, but not so many that they need to be in the hospital-like setting of an LTACH.

Skilled Nursing Facility

Patients who can benefit from some rehab and assistance with everyday activities live in a skilled nursing facility (SNF). This is also known as a nursing home. If the patient does not have enough support at home, this may be recommended over home health.

Home Health

Patients who are healthy enough to return home but are not safe to travel may benefit from home health. Therapists come to the home to work with the patient. This may be preferred to a SNF if other people are available to care for the patient at home.

Outpatient Rehabilitation

Some patients can return home and are able to safely travel to rehab. This is referred to as outpatient rehabilitation.

One or more of these facilities may be needed before a patient can return to their desired way of life. There may not be much choice of which level of care the patient needs, but there may be a choice of which rehab facility to use. By comparing the different facilities, the patient and family can choose the best for them. This can be done on the Centers for Medicare and Medicaid Services website (link available at NavigatingTheICU.com). It may also help to tour the facility and speak with other residents.

Nurse's Note

- Recovery is a physical and emotional workout for the patient. Realizing the long-term effects of the illness, such as physical and mental limitations, lifestyle changes, and rehab requirements, is tough. Try to prepare everyone for a realistic recovery by asking the medical team for their opinion.
- The patient's attitude and motivation make a big difference. Try to encourage your loved one as much as possible and remind them why they are putting in the hard work.
- Encourage your loved one to be as independent as possible in rehab so they can develop the skills to leave.
- As soon as possible, begin planning for the patient's transfer out of the hospital. Talk to the case manager or discharge planner about what options are best for the patient and family.
- Support groups, found online or through the medical team, can be helpful to see what rehab is like, learn tips for success, and choose the best facility.
- Many hospitals have online resources for patients that have personalized and important information, such as their diagnosis, medications, follow-up appointments, ways to contact their providers, etc. It may be called a patient portal, and this is a great way to keep track of your medical past, present, and future. You may have to ask the nurse to explain the process of activating the account.

Questions to Ask the ICU Team About Leaving the Hospital

- What are the patient's needs going to be after leaving the hospital?
- What is the timeframe for the patient's likely recovery?
- What do you think the most difficult parts will be with the patient's goals of care in mind?
- How could the patient's daily life be affected by post-intensive care syndrome?
- What are good resources or support groups for the patient and family?

Resource

Next Steps in Care is a website with valuable information for families and patients for when the time comes to transfer out of the ICU (link available at NavigatingTheICU.com).

13

Common Concerns and Helpful Tips

This chapter discusses some common concerns that patients and families have in the intensive care unit (ICU). From mentioning small tips that can make a big difference, to describing life-changing situations, this section helps answer questions, explains what to expect, and gives some advice that patients and families might not know. As with the other chapters, the medical staff may have much to add to these topics.

What to Bring to the Hospital and What to Leave at Home

If someone has an illness, it may be worth developing a plan for how to get to medical care quickly. Creating a list of things to bring to the hospital, or organizing a prepacked bag can be helpful for this stressful situation. Below is a list of items patients and families appreciate during a hospital stay.

- Need a prepacked bag to quickly grab on the way out the door?
  - List of medications (prescriptions, vitamins, and supplements), dosages, and how often they are taken
  - Perscribed medications
  - List of medical history (past illnesses, surgeries, current issues, and allergies)

- List of phone numbers for family, friends, and current providers (if not in phone)
- Identification and insurance information
- Advance care planning documents (advance directive, living will, durable power of attorney [DPOA] for healthcare, etc)
- Glasses, dentures, hearing aids with batteries, and their containers
- Phone and charger
- Headphones
- Photos, books, magazines, and coloring books
- Lip balm
- Fan
- Favorite pillow or blanket
- Sleeping mask and carplugs
- Snacks (not for patient)
- Leave unnecessary jewelry, cash, over-the-counter medications, and other valuables at home.

Nurse's Note

In case you will not be able to take care of your usual responsibilities due to your illness, you may want to make a backup plan. For instance, you may not be able to pay your bills, feed your pet, etc. To make sure your affairs are in order, you can create a list or phone note that details important things. Then, you can let a trusted family member or friend know about this list. Some important considerations are when bills need to be paid, where keys, titles, and other important assests are located, necessary legal and financial points of contact, login and passwords for online accounts, pets and plants to take care of, etc.

How to Make the ICU Stay More Comfortable

The ICU prioritizes saving lives over everyday comforts. However, there are some things found in many ICUs that can make the stay more enjoyable:

- Warm blanket
- Pillows
- Socks
- Television channel list
- Relaxing TV channel with calming music

- Room phone
- Video calling
- Cafeteria menu
- Nutritional drinks (Ensure, Glucerna), diet soda, sandwiches, graham crackers, peanut butter, Jell-O, pudding, ice cream, and popsicles
- Skin moisturizer
- Lip balm or mouth moisturizer
- Toothbrush and toothpaste
- Warmed, rinse-free shampoo cap
- Ear plugs and eye mask
- Headphones
- Air freshener
- Do Not Disturb order—allows a stable patient more undisturbed time overnight
- Possible medications the provider can order: eye drops, cough medicine, spray to numb the throat, special lotion for itchy skin, natural sleep aid, antinausea medication, gas relief, and heartburn medication
- Those who use tobacco can request a nicotine patch (however, this may be a great time to quit the habit)
- Spiritual services
- Therapy animals, music therapy, and other similar comforts may be available—check with the nurse

For families:

- Many hospitals can recommend nearby hotels that discount rooms for families of patients.
- A meal for family members may be a possibility.

How to Communicate With the ICU Team

The best results depend on a trusting relationship between the patient, family, and medical team. Open, honest, and respectful communication helps to build this relationship. Understandably, many patients and families can feel unsure, overwhelmed, or hesitant to bring issues up to the medical staff. However, the family knows the patient best. So, they may be able to recognize something important before the ICU team. Therefore, it can be helpful to know the best ways to bring something to the attention of the staff.

Typically, the nurse is the best staff member to approach because they have the most contact with the patient. It is best to bring up any concerns in the morning to the nurse. If necessary, the nurse can then address the issues during the morning rounds.

During this time, the entire team is present to listen and make a plan. If the issue arises after rounds, the family can relay this to the nurse. The nurse may be able to solve the problem directly. If the family needs to speak with the providers, the nurse knows the best ways to contact them.

It is worth thinking if the issue requires a discussion. If the family wants to update the team about something simple, such as unrelieved patient pain, this can be brought to the nurse. If it is a more in-depth issue, such as needing an update on the patient's overall plan, it may be worth meeting with the provider. Some situations need an in-depth discussion with many ICU team members, such as when deciding the goals of care for a very sick patient. This discussion benefits from the experience of the medical team and family. In this type of situation, the family should ask the nurse to set up a family meeting with the medical team.

Below are some general tips and phrasing suggestions for communicating with the medical team.

- Try to:
  - Begin by asking the staff member to speak when they have a free moment.
  - Bring up all of the concerns at one time, starting with the most important.
  - Create a list of questions or concerns to give to a member of the medical team.
  - Mention why the issue is important and how it will benefit the patient.
  - Use your resources, such as the nurse, provider, social worker, etc.
  - Treat the staff the way you want to be treated.
  - Thank the team for caring for the patient.
- Try not to:
  - Bring up a concern while the staff is in the middle of patient care.
  - Blame anyone.

Phrasing that might be helpful:

"When you have a moment, I was wondering if you thought this might be important..."
"I know you are very busy, but it would make the patient's day if ...."
"We are concerned because, although the care has been great, this is worrying because ...."
"What's the best way to clear up ...."
"Who's the best person to talk to about ...."

Not Allowed to Eat or Drink—Nil Per Os (NPO)

If a patient has trouble swallowing or has a procedure requiring sedation, they may be placed under a <u>NPO</u> order (nil per os, meaning "nothing by mouth" in Latin). This means the patient cannot have anything to eat or drink. Usually, this is to prevent food or liquid from getting into the lungs, known as aspiration. How long the patient needs to be NPO depends on the reason, but they are allowed to eat and drink once it is safe. During this time, the patient's blood sugar is checked regularly to make sure it is normal. Also, essential medications are still given, and IV fluids may be started to keep the patient hydrated. The family can confirm these with the medical team.

Understandably, being NPO can bother patients. Luckily, there are ways to ease the discomfort. The nurse may be able to give moistened swabs to wet the patient's mouth. In some cases, the patient can suck on ice chips for relief. Additionally, lip balm or mouth moisturizer can be helpful. Sometimes, thirsty patients are just hot. Placing a cool, wet towel on their forehead and reducing the room temperature can help. Also, an icepack on the neck may relieve thirst. As with many discomforts, distraction with TV, movies, phone calls, books, etc, can be effective.

Nurse's Note

- If you are NPO for a procedure and it gets to be late in the day, ask if the procedure is still going to take place. If not, ask to have your diet changed so you can eat.
- A procedure scheduled for later in the day may allow for a breakfast of clear liquids (Jell-O, broth, juice, popsicles, etc). You can ask if this is possible and when the latest you can eat is.

Unable to Visit the Patient

Sometimes it is not possible to visit a family member in the hospital. It may be too far to travel in a short amount of time. Or, hospitals may not allow visitors in order to limit the spread of diseases. Whatever the reason, families can still be a presence at the bedside. This section mentions some other possibilities when visiting in person is not an option.

The first step is to understand the visitation policy. Please see Visiting the Patient, page 17.

A quick way to get updated on the patient's recent progress and the plan for the day is to call the nurse. The nurse can answer questions and connect the caller to the patient or other members of the medical team. Please be mindful that the beginning of the shift is busy (7:00 AM and 7:00 PM), and the nurse may not be able to provide updates around these times. The best way to get the most out of an update is by planning a time or two with the nurse. Usually, around 10:00 AM, 2:00 PM, and 10:00 PM are less busy.

It is also important to narrow down who will be calling. Understandably, many concerned family members want updates and unknowingly flood the nurse with calls. Problematically, all the time spent updating the many family members takes away from the available time to care for the patient. This is the nurse's first priority and is more important than updating family. Unfortunately, the family can then feel ignored because the busy nurse cannot quickly return the calls. Additionally, repeating information to many family members increases the risk of miscommunications within the family, which leads to other issues.

To reduce these problems, it is best if one person, usually the spouse or next of kin, receives the updates and communicates the news with the rest of the family. This person can then decide who else should hear the information.

Nurse's Note

- Please do not call during shift change, usually 7:00 AM and 7:00 PM. These are the times when the oncoming nurse is learning about the patient from the offgoing nurse. Any interruptions can result in missed information and affect patient safety.
- If anything major changes, the medical team will give you a call.

A video call allows the family to be at the bedside virtually, and patients tend to enjoy it. This can be scheduled when calling for an update. Please confirm the best way to video call (Skype, FaceTime, Zoom, etc), the right number to call, and a time that works for the nurse and the family. There may be a limit on the duration and number of video calls to allow the patient to rest and others to use the device.

Nurse's Note

- I have seen many distressed family members spend a fortune and make huge sacrifices to get to the bedside on short notice. Video calls are a valuable substitute. Many family members can join, the timing is flexible, and it is convenient and safe.

An additional benefit of video calling is the ability to schedule family meetings with the medical team. It can be difficult to gather important family members and the medical team together at one time. The family meeting on video call is a convenient way to introduce everyone, discuss important questions, and make plans. It helps to have questions ready and focus the conversation to make sure it is valuable for everyone.

Strategies for Reducing the Costs of Treatment

A common concern for patients and families is the cost of medical treatment. Because of this, hospitals are familiar with how to address this issue without affecting the quality of the care they provide. Importantly, the patient or family must speak up if they want costs to be addressed.

When admitted to the ICU, the patient or family can relay to the medical team their concern over the costs of procedures, medicine, etc. The best people to say this to are the provider, nurse, social worker, and case manager. Additionally, someone from the hospital's billing department will contact the patient or their family to determine the patient's insurance. This is another good time to mention a desire to discuss ways to reduce costs. They might be able to reduce the price of care in two ways.

The first way for savings is through the hospital's billing department, which provides patients and their families with cost-related information. They can be asked for tips to reduce hospital expenses. For example, because the patient is charged many times during ICU treatment, asking for an itemized bill can help patients make sure they are paying only for what was used. If any mistakes were made, the billing department can correct them.

In some cases, families simply are not able to pay the requested amount. If families contact the billing department, it may be able to reduce the bill. This department also provides payment plans to make payment easier. The patient's social worker and case manager can also ask the billing department about this request.

The second opportunity for savings is the medical team's ability to prescribe less expensive medications. Sometimes there are different medications, called generic, that cost less and work just as well. The pharmacist or provider know which of these are best for the patient. The social worker or case manager can recommend the best way to get these medications when the patient leaves the hospital.

The patient and family should ask the provider or pharmacist if all of the medications they are prescribed are needed. This is especially true for the medicine prescribed before the current hospitalization. In some cases, it may make sense to switch to a nonprescription medication. Another option may be to split in half a double-strength pill. Then, taking the half-pill would be the correct dose. Importantly, the first step is to talk with the medical staff about how these expenses are affecting you.

The social worker and case manager work with patients and their family to help the patient continue to recover after the hospital stay. They know the resources around the patient's home that are most helpful. They also know the best tips for reducing costs. Before patients leave the hospital, they should make a plan with the social worker and case manager for using those services. Also, a plan should be made for how to follow up with them after leaving the hospital in case questions arise.

Nurse's Note

■ An important part of saving costs is prevention. If you or your loved one can prevent accidents or illnesses, money can be saved. For instance, prevent a fall and broken bone by working on your strength and coordination now with physical therapy and occupational therapy. Prevent an illness by finding reliable ways to take your medicine. The medical team can provide you with resources and tips to do this. The more you can avoid the need for healthcare, the more money you can save.

■ There is funding for medical care. Please see NavigatingTheICU.com for the links.

Questions to Ask When Making a Decision

Unfortunately, patients can become sicker in the ICU. When this happens, just understanding the situation can be hard. What makes this moment even harder is that, after learning the bad news, a decision needs to be made for the medical care. To decide what the next steps should be, the right information is needed. Below is a list of questions that can help gather the right information to make the best decision. Although any of the medical staff can be asked, the provider who directs the medical care, is the best resource. Sometimes, more information can be overwhelming. Therefore, the most important questions to ask are in **bold**.

- What problem occurred and in what part of the body?
- What has already been done to help the problem?
- Is more information needed (labs, tests, imaging, etc)?
- **Why is medical help needed?**
- **What are the options for treatment that align with the patient's goals of care?**
  - Procedure vs. medicine vs. wait and see vs. combination?
- For each option:
  - **What is the most likely outcome for similar patients?**
  - **What is the best-case scenario and how common is it?**
  - **What is the worst-case scenario and how common is it?**
  - **How is the patient recovery and family experience in the short and long term?**
  - How often do the risks happen during and after?
- What do both the patient and family need to think about moving forward?
- **When does a decision need to be made?**

Nurse's Note

- Even the best, most experienced medical team may not know exactly how a patient will recover. Sometimes, only the best guess can be provided. Please do not be frustrated or lose confidence in the medical team. Rather, this is a sign of honest and open communication so everyone involved can be on the same page. This way, everyone can work together to make the best decision.

- It is OK to ask what the medical team's recommendation is. Combining the patient's goals with the medical team's knowledge of treatments can help produce the best plan of care.

- It can help to have another person present to remember what is said, ask questions, and provide moral support.

- These questions are repeated in Appendix 4, page 185, with space to write down the information.

Second Opinion

A second opinion, when a different provider examines the patient, can be a valuable option. This provider is separate from the main ICU team. They work on their own to determine the patient's illness (diagnosis), the patient's likely recovery (prognosis), and the available treatment options. For those with a rare disease or life-threatening illness, or those who may require surgery or complex treatment, a second opinion can confirm the current plan or offer other options.

Second opinions are common in medicine, and the medical team should be supportive. This request can be made through the ICU team or with another hospital. Virtual second opinions are also an option. This is when another provider electronically assesses the patient and their medical information. Importantly, the patient and family should make it clear to the new provider which questions they want answered with the second opinion. These questions should match the patient's goals of care. For instance, is the family wondering what all of the options for treatment are, so they can make a plan that is in line with the patient's goals of care? This way, the medical team and family can work together to make the best decision for the patient.

Although this information can be valuable, time may be limited in the ICU. A second opinion may not be an option if the illness is immediately life threatening. Quick action to save the patient's life may be more important than more information.

When there is enough time for a second opinion, patients and families commonly say it makes them feel better. Sometimes, the second opinion can change a diagnosis or offer other options for treatment. Even if it does not change anything, knowing that all options were explored can reduce guilt or doubt.

Nurse's Note

- It is best to request a second opinion as soon as you know you want one because the patient's health can change quickly in the ICU.
- When choosing who will provide the second opinion, you want someone who is an <u>expert</u> in the illness and is <u>experienced</u>.
- Check with your insurance if a second or third opinion is covered.
- When both opinions agree, choose the provider based on your gut feeling.
- If they disagree, choose the option that matches the patient's goals of care most. You may be able to ask the providers to discuss the case while you listen to determine whose advice to follow.

Full Code and Do Not Attempt Resuscitation

Desired Treatments If the Heart Stops

Any stay in the ICU should involve a discussion about which treatments the patient wants if their heart stops. This decision is selecting between being "full code" or "do not attempt resuscitate." The patient has to decide which is best, depending on their goals of care (page 135).

A full code patient wants everything done if their heart stops. If this happens, the ICU team works to restore a healthy heartbeat. This is attempted by pushing on the chest (chest compressions), inserting a breathing tube, giving medications, and shocking the patient's heart. This is called a "code blue," which is discussed in the next section.

A code blue attempts to restart the heart. It does not cure what caused the heart to stop. At best, if the heart is restarted, the patient is still as sick as they were before. Furthermore, a code blue may cause injuries, such as broken ribs from chest compressions. It also may not prevent organ damage or death. For instance, brain injury can occur from low oxygen levels while the heart was stopped. This may result in permanent disability. Recovering without lasting injury is rare. However, some patients do make a full recovery.

Some patients decide that, if their heart stops, they do not want therapy to restart it. This is called do not attempt resuscitation or do not resuscitate (DNR). Some reasons for choosing to be DNR include the patient's satisfaction with the life they have lived, acceptance of eventual death, a willingness to let nature take its course, or a desire to not experience a code blue and the potential resulting disabilities. Importantly, if their heart stops, they can still receive medicine to make them comfortable.

The patient can also choose any combination of the four options: breathing tube, chest compressions, medications, and shocking the heart. However, for the best chance to regain a healthy heartbeat, all four are needed. Whatever the choice, the patient's preference will be followed. Additionally, this decision can be changed later. However, it needs to be discussed with the provider for it to take effect and be entered into the patient's medical record.

Nurse's Note

- Please do not be alarmed if this is discussed early in your, or your loved one's, hospital stay. The medical team wants to make sure the patient's desires are followed.

- Some patients think that full code means full care and that DNR means less care. This is not true. This decision only applies if the patient's heart stops. Everything before that will be full, aggressive treatment for both full code and DNR patients.

- Another option is to discuss with the medical team what the likelihood of a full recovery would be if your heart stopped in your present health. Depending on your illness, you may have a better or worse chance of recovering after a code blue. You could then decide whether going through the code blue would be worth it.

- Some patients are OK going through the code blue and then allowing their durable power of attorney (DPOA) to decide whether to continue treatment based on their potential for recovery. Please see Goals of Care, page 135, for tips when discussing this with your DPOA.

What Happens If the Heart Stops for a Full Code Patient (Code Blue)

When a full code patient's heart stops, the ICU team follows a plan that tries to restart a healthy heartbeat, called Advanced Cardiovascular Life Support (ACLS). This is similar to cardiopulmonary resuscitation (CPR). During this time, the patient is "coding" and a "code blue" is occurring.

At the moment the heart stops, the patient is dead. The medical team will try to bring them back to life.

During a code blue, many actions occur quickly. The first is chest compressions, where someone pushes down on the patient's chest repeatedly. This squeezes the heart to pump blood around the body. The code alarm may ring, which notifies the medical team that help is needed. Many staff enter the room to do other jobs. If not already in place, a breathing tube is inserted as chest compressions continue. Two sticky pads are placed on the chest to try to shock the heart back to a healthy heartbeat. Also, all patients who code receive epinephrine, a medication that attempts to restart the heart. The medication and shocks are given at planned times according to

ACLS. Other treatments may be given to try to reverse the cause of the stopped heart.

A code blue can last anywhere from minutes to hours. It stops when a healthy heartbeat returns, or when the leading provider determines that nothing more can be done for the patient. Sometimes, patients can code more than once in a short amount of time.

Although the family does not help with the code blue, they usually can watch. Many ICU staff encourage family to stay so the process of trying to bring the patient back to life is seen. If the patient cannot be revived, the family can see that everything possible was tried. Understandably, many families choose to wait outside the room.

What Happens After Surviving a Code Blue

If a healthy heartbeat is restored, the medical team tries to prevent the heart from stopping again. They investigate the reasons why the patient's heart stopped and try to fix them. The medical team also follows guidelines to, hopefully, save the patient's organs. This is done by keeping their oxygen and blood pressure at normal levels, which may require medication or procedures.

Depending on how long the heart was stopped, there may have been time when the brain and other organs were not receiving oxygen—a condition known as <u>anoxia</u>. If oxygen levels in the body were low, the organs could have been hurt. Blood tests can tell if they are damaged. When an organ is so damaged that the body cannot function normally, it is called failure. At this point, the patient needs medical care to assist or replace that organ. For instance, a patient with kidney failure needs dialysis for the body to function normally.

If the patient is not acting the same as before the code, brain damage may have occurred. To limit this damage, the patient is cooled. Their temperature is lowered to 89.6 to 93.2°F. This is known as <u>targeted temperature management</u> or therapeutic hypothermia. Usually this lasts for 24 to 48 hours. Once the patient is returned to a normal temperature, the ICU team can see if brain injury has occurred.

After a code, immediate and long-term treatment plans should be developed for the patient's probable recovery. The plans should include what that recovery looks like for the patient and family in the months and years ahead.

These moments are difficult. The uncertainty of recovery is stressful. Positive strides can be made that encourage optimism, and setbacks can follow that are devastating.

In these moments, the family must use their resources. Of course, nurses are available to discuss the immediate plan for the patient or connect the family to other resources. Additionally, a meeting can be arranged with the medical team if updates are needed or the plan needs to be discussed. Spiritual services can be helpful in these difficult times. Social workers are also skilled at discussing issues commonly facing families in this situation, and they know how to access the resources that are most helpful. Often the hardest part of this process is waiting and feeling helpless. Acknowledging this and committing effort in these other ways can help to reduce this emotional weight. Please see Chapters 10 and 11 for more ideas (page 102 and page 105) for more ideas.

Nurse's Note

- Whether you are deciding between full code and not attempt resuscitation, wondering what care you would want if you were unable to choose, or directing care for someone who cannot respond, Chapter 14 can help give you direction, page 135.

What Happens If a Patient May Be Having a Stroke (Code Stroke)

Every medical professional is trained to look for the signs of a stroke. A stroke, known as a cerebrovascular accident, is when a part of the brain is starved of oxygen. Without oxygen, the brain tissue dies. This can happen in two ways. The first way is when a blocked blood vessel prevents blood flow and oxygen from reaching part of the brain. This is called an ischemic stroke. The second way is when a broken blood vessel leaks blood within the skull. As the amount of blood builds up, it squeezes part of the brain. This prevents blood flow and oxygen from reaching that area. This is called a hemorrhagic stroke.

The resulting brain damage changes how a person normally acts or controls their body. These changes signal that a stroke is happening. Recognizing a stroke quickly is important because the faster it is identified, the sooner treatment can begin to save the brain.

A helpful tool to recognize a stroke is "BE FAST," which is also a reminder that speed is important. Each letter stands for some of the common signs of a stroke. Remember, these are all <u>sudden</u> changes from the patient's normal appearance or behavior.

- **B**alance—Is there a loss of balance?
- **E**yes—Is there loss of vision?
- **F**ace—Is the face uneven or is one side droopy?
- **A**rms—Is there uneven strength in the arms or legs, or is one side numb?
- **S**peech—Is the speech slurred or hard to produce? Are random words being said that make no sense?
- **T**errible headache—Is there a terrible headache?

All of these symptoms reflect one critical point: There is a sudden change in the patient's appearance or behavior. Outside of the hospital, 911 should be called immediately. If a sign of a stroke appears in the ICU, a "code stroke" is called.

A <u>code stroke</u> is designed to identify a brain injury and begin treatment as soon as possible. After it is called, a brain-focused medical team springs into action with a stroke-focused checklist. A provider trained in evaluating brain function assesses the patient. Blood sugar levels are confirmed to be normal, as a low level can cause symptoms similar to a stroke. Medication and oxygen may be given. Pictures of the patient's brain are taken with a computed tomography (CT) scan or magnetic resonance imaging (MRI) to see if there is a blockage or a bleed in the brain. Recommendations are then made for the best plan moving forward.

Nurse's Note

- Write down the time when the patient changed. This will determine what treatments are possible.
- Do not allow the patient to eat, drink, or take medication. These could make the illness worse.
- Do not allow the patient to get out of bed unless the nurse is present. Your loved one could fall and hurt themselves.

Figure 13.1 Functions of the Brain

Each section, or lobe, of the brain is in charge of different functions. When a lobe is injured, that function is impaired.

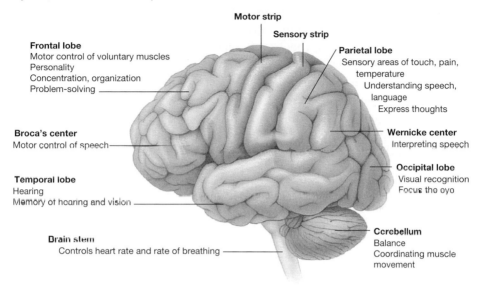

Motor strip

Sensory strip

Frontal lobe
Motor control of voluntary muscles
Personality
Concentration, organization
Problem-solving

Parietal lobe
Sensory areas of touch, pain, temperature
Understanding speech, language
Express thoughts

Broca's center
Motor control of speech

Wernicke center
Interpreting speech

Occipital lobe
Visual recognition
Focus the eye

Temporal lobe
Hearing
Memory of hearing and vision

Cerebellum
Balance
Coordinating muscle movement

Brain stem
Controls heart rate and rate of breathing

The Most Serious Types of Brain Injury

The most serious brain injuries result in a loss of awareness. Generally, this means the patient cannot interact with anyone or anything. The three most serious types of brain injury are a vegetative state, a coma, and brain death. Common causes of these are low oxygen levels and physical injury (trauma) to the brain. Understanding these categories can help the family make decisions. Questions about survival and recovery should be discussed with the medical team.

A <u>vegetative state</u>, also called unresponsive wakefulness syndrome, can be disturbing for the family because the patient appears to be awake. For instance, their eyes may be open and blinking, they may fall asleep at night, and they may yawn or cry. Worryingly, they may even react to something painful. These actions indicate their reflexes work, and the part of their brain that controls basic functions is alive. For instance, their breathing, heart rate, and blood pressure are usually normal. However, there is no evidence that they are aware of themselves. Importantly, they cannot interact with other people or with objects. They do not respond to commands or attempt to communicate.

Similar to a vegetative state, a patient in a <u>coma</u> is unaware of themselves and shows no signs of interaction. However, a comatose patient differs because they do not appear to be awake. They do not open their eyes, and they rarely react to something painful. They may have basic reflexes, such as a cough or gag, and they might breathe on their own. Typically, patients with brain injury do not stay in a coma longer than a few weeks. They recover, die, or progress into a vegetative state. In some cases, brain death occurs.

<u>Brain death</u> is when a patient looks like they are in a coma, except they lack the reflexes needed to live. For example, this patient cannot breathe on their own, so they need a breathing tube. They may also have trouble controlling their heart rate and blood pressure, so these functions may require medical support. There is no recovering from brain death, and this patient is considered legally dead.

There are many tests that can show the health of the brain. One way is to test the patient's reflexes. The following reflexes show that the basic functions of the brain are working:

- Pupils—Shining a light in the eyes to see if the pupils constrict (get smaller).
- Gag—Inserting a suction catheter to see if the patient gags.
- Cough—Inserting a suction catheter to see if the patient coughs.
- Corneal—Brushing the eyelashes to see if the eyelid moves.
- Oculocephalic—Turning the head to one side to see if the eyes move in the opposite direction.

An additional brain function test is the <u>apnea test</u>. The ICU team temporarily pauses the breaths provided by the ventilator. If the patient does not breathe on their own, this is an indication that brain death has occurred. Another option is to have an <u>electroencephalography</u> (EEG) test. This test measures brain waves through electrodes on different areas of the scalp. Stimulation (light flashes, pain, sound, etc) causes brain wave responses in healthy patients. Those who are brain dead do not have these responses. Some providers may recommend brain imaging to determine brain death. For instance, there are tests that can track the blood flow in the brain. No blood flow indicates brain death. Before and after these tests, discussions with the medical team should detail what is happening, what degree of recovery is likely, and what needs to be done moving forward.

There are some reflexes that can give family members false hope. One is the Lazarus reflex, where patients with brain death move their arms up to their chest. Another is a triple flexion, where a leg, when stimulated, pulls toward the body. These reflexes only require the patient to have a healthy spinal cord. Unfortunately, they do not show brain function or recovery.

Nurse's Note

▪ There is some overlap between these three types of brain injury. To ensure you are making the best decisions, a discussion should occur with a provider familiar with brain injury. Please see Appendix 4, page 185, for an outline of questions to ask.

A Quick Guide to Organ Donation

The moments surrounding organ donation can be difficult for the family. Without a doubt, organ donation saves lives. But this fact can be of small comfort to those losing a loved one. The ICU staff and the organ recipients thank the patient and their family for the decision to be a donor.

If all of the organs are healthy, one donor can potentially save eight lives. Each of the lungs, both kidneys, the heart, pancreas, small intestines, and liver are the organs that can be received. Tissues can also be donated, such as heart valves and corneas. There are always more people who need organs and tissues than are available.

There are some common myths of organ donation. One is that organ donors do not receive the same medical treatment as nondonors. The reality is that the decision to be a donor does not affect medical treatment. Patients and family should be aware that donors and nondonors will receive equal, aggressive medical care. It is only after confirming that the patient has no chance of recovery that donation is considered. Another myth is that organ donation prevents an open-casket funeral. The reality is that, throughout the donation process, care is taken to ensure this will be possible. Any concerns can be directed to the donation organization. This organization guides the entire process, including matching the donor with the recipient.

By law, the decision to be a donor is the patient's choice. Usually, this decision is made when renewing a driver's license or by signing up online. These agreements count as consent. If the choice has not been made, the donation organization contacts the person who makes decisions for the patient, the DPOA. The DPOA then decides if the patient will be a potential donor. This conversation only happens if the patient is very sick and cannot make their own decisions.

The ability to be a donor depends on the patient's medical history and current illness. What matters most is that the organs are healthy. Also, medical advances are changing the possibilities for donating and receiving organs. For instance, HIV used to disqualify patients from being donors. However, organs from these patients are now accepted by some recipients. The donation organization decides which organs can potentially be donated. This occurs only after it is determined that the patient has no chance of recovery.

A common donor patient has a brain injury that results in brain death. This patient cannot get better. However, the patient's organs are healthy, and the body is supported with machines and medicine. The decision to pursue donation is discussed only after confirming that the patient has no chance of recovery and is a donor. The donation organization then contacts the DPOA about the donation. The donation organization explains the process and answers any questions. The patient may need to have tests done to see how healthy the organs are.

Before the donation begins, the family has time to say good-bye. Then, the patient is taken to the operating room where surgery to remove the organs begins. Throughout this time the ICU team is available for any questions and to support the family.

Nurse's Note

- Please do not be offended if the ICU team directs donation questions to the donation organization. This organization knows the whole process well and can give you more specific information.
- Some donation organizations allow the donor family to communicate with the organ recipient after the transplant. This can be a bright spot in difficult times. If this interests you, mention it to the donation organization.

14

Critical Questions That Determine the Right Care

Goals of Care

What Amount of Medical Therapy Is Right for The Patient?

The patient's medical care should try to produce abilities that are desired and realistic. These abilities then create an acceptable quality of life. This is the goal of each procedure, test, and medication that the intensive care unit (ICU) team recommends. Tailoring medical therapy to suit the patient's preferences for their life is known as the goals of care or goals of medical care. For example, many patients say they want everything done to stay alive. Because of this, the medical team tries all life-sustaining options to achieve this goal. It should be noted that trying all life-sustaining options occurs automatically unless the patient states otherwise.

The patient's goals of care may shift over the course of an illness. One way this can happen is when the patient's potential to meet their goal changes. **For instance, say that a patient named Sarah values eating meals with her family for a good quality of life. This is a cherished time of connection with those she loves most Unfortunately, an illness brings Sarah into the ICU and prevents her ability to safely eat food. If she eats and chokes, she may develop a deadly lung infection. This could jeopardize what she values most, sharing meals with her family.** In this case, the ICU team and patient need to work together to identify a different goal that is desirable and realistic. The medical care is then adjusted to assist the patient toward the new abilities. **Sarah and the ICU team agree on a feeding tube for nutrition in the hopes that she will regain the ability to eat soon. Although Sarah cannot enjoy food, she still cherishes the ability to spend time with her family when they visit the ICU.**

Another possible shift in the goals of care occurs when too much time or too many procedures are needed to recover desired abilities. If the patient's path to recovery lengthens, the amount of medical treatment wanted may change. In this case, "everything" may not be the right plan. **For instance, say Sarah's recovery is slow. As a result, the ICU team believes that she will need the feeding tube for much longer. However, Sarah misses sharing meals with her family. This is important to her quality of life. Therefore, she decides that she does not want to wait until she might be able to eat safely. Sarah wants to eat now even though she knows that food may get into her lungs and worsen her illness.** The patient and ICU team then work together to form a new plan that matches the new goal. **Sarah and the ICU team agree that eating soft foods slowly can give her the satisfaction of sharing meals with her family while lowering the risk of a lung infection.** Communication and trust between the patient and ICU team are essential for this process to work well.

Over the entire course of the ICU stay, the goals of care need to be revisited because things can change for better and for worse. If the goals change, they need to be shared with the ICU team. The discussions about the patient's probable recovery, their preferences for life, and how to achieve their desired abilities are essential. This process is called shared decision making. It combines the patient's goals with the ICU team's knowledge of medical options to make the best plan.

Advance Care Planning

Desired Medical Therapies If the Ability to Choose Is Absent

Making decisions about which medical care would be preferred in different situations is called <u>advance care planning</u>. Advance care planning is documented with <u>advance directives</u>. These are legal documents that tell what medical care someone wants if they are unable to make decisions. There are many forms of advance directives, such as the durable power of attorney, living will, and physician orders for life-sustaining treatment.

Durable Power of Attorney

Who Will Make Decisions for the Patient?

The durable power of attorney (DPOA), also known as a proxy or surrogate, is the legal term for the person who makes medical decisions for the patient if the patient cannot. Importantly, this is different than a financial DPOA. If the patient has not chosen a DPOA, depending on state law, it usually follows the next of kin by default. The spouse is first considered to be the legal DPOA, if capable and willing, followed by the adult child, etc.

In the ICU, there are many reasons why a patient would not be able to choose their medical care. This can be due to the injury or illness that brought the patient to the ICU, the effects of medication, or ongoing medical care that limits communication. When it is determined that the patient lacks capacity (the ability to understand and communicate their choice, page 23), the DPOA becomes the decision-maker. However, if the patient regains capacity at any time, the patient can then make their own decisions.

The responsibility of the DPOA is a challenging and honorable service to someone in need. The DPOA has to set aside personal expectations and desires to make tough medical decisions that the patient would have wanted. It can be very difficult. Importantly, a discussion has to occur between the patient and their DPOA to ensure the necessary information is known. This makes potential medical decisions clearer for the DPOA. Tips for this conversation are outlined in the following sections.

Provided below are some guidelines for choosing an ideal DPOA.

Durable Power of Attorney—Someone to make medical decisions for you if you are incapacitated.

- Choose someone you can trust to ask difficult questions and make hard, thoughtful decisions.
- Choose someone who will work with the ICU team for your specific medical care requests and/or to produce your desired abilities for an acceptable quality of life.
- Be aware of who your DPOA is by default and change if necessary.
- Must be at least 18 years old.
- Ask their permission to be your DPOA.
- Discuss your living will with your DPOA (see Living Will, page 139, and Goal of Living Until Death, page 142).

- Make this decision known (the process depends on your state).
  - Make the DPOA official legally.
  - Consider uploading the document to an online registry so it can be easily accessed if needed.
  - Give copies to your doctors and bring one to the hospital.
  - See NavigatingTheICU.com for helpful resources.

Nurse's Note

- Selecting a DPOA is the <u>most important decision</u> for securing your wishes in the event you cannot participate. Your DPOA can change your explicit requests, such as what is outlined in your living will. Therefore, choosing the right person is essential.
- Sometimes, the DPOA by default is <u>NOT</u> the best choice to carry out your wishes. Find out who is your automatic DPOA and change it if necessary.
- You may be able to choose a second DPOA in case the first is not available when needed. See your state's rules for details.
- If you have concerns or would like to update this document, please ask your nurse to connect you with the appropriate ICU representative. You may be able to update it during the current hospitalization.

Responsibilities When Making Decisions for the Patient

A Message to the Durable Power of Attorney

You, as the DPOA, have three important and honorable commitments. The first commitment is to discuss with the patient the medical care they would want and for how long they would be willing to try to achieve their goals. This should occur as soon as possible, ideally before any medical care is needed. Furthermore, this discussion needs to be repeated if any abilities are lost and after significant life changes. Please refer to Living Will, page 139, and Goal of Living Until Death, page 142, as a guide.

The second commitment is to honor the patient's wishes in their moment of need. There is no better way to respect your loved one and preserve their dignity than by fulfilling their medical desires. You are enabling them to live and die according to their cherished values. You are empowering someone who is powerless.

The third commitment is to treat yourself with respect and kindness. Take care of yourself as much as possible. Choosing medical therapies for another is hard, especially when they are based on complex medical information. You are asked to make life-changing decisions about a loved one that may have uncertain consequences. Anxiety, doubt, and stress are common, even when the best way forward is known. Unfortunately, other factors can make this time more challenging, such as financial issues and disagreeing family members. Please refer to Chapter 10 (page 102) and Chapter 11 (page 105) for suggestions about how to best treat yourself and your loved one.

Nurse's Note

- You are not alone in making decisions. Family and friends can be supportive if they put the patient's desires first. Within the ICU, helpful resources are the social worker, nurse, spiritual services, provider, and ethics committee.

- Asking for a goals of care meeting, also known as a family meeting, can help resolve conflict and unify those who disagree. During this meeting, the ICU team and family gather to agree on a plan that is best for the patient (page 147).

- If this position is not right for you, you can decline to be the DPOA. This shows respect for yourself and the patient, and it is OK. This is also better than not making any decisions. Please ask the ICU team if you have questions about this.

- If your loved one is incapacitated and without an advance directive, use the sections, Living Will, page 139, and Goal of Living Until Death, page 142, to think about what they would want. Did your loved one ever discuss situations like this with you, your friends, or family? What was their reaction like? Was it positive or negative? The next sections can help guide your thoughts about what your loved one may have preferred. The section, If the Patient Cannot Respond, page 147, discusses how you can work with the ICU team to decide on the best plan for the patient.

Living Will

How to Choose Medical Therapies Now in Case Decisions Cannot Be Made Later

A living will outlines the medical care a patient wants to receive or refuse if they are unable to make this decision when needed. The patient chooses their preferred medical care and life support measures for different illnesses or situations. The requests can be as general or specific as desired, but more information can help make the decisions of the DPOA easier.

A living will has limits. One problem is that a patient may not know how each medical treatment would affect their ability to enjoy life. So, they may be unable to confidently judge if they would want it. A living will also cannot outline the preferences for every possible illness and potential recovery. Additionally, it needs to be updated when the patient's desires change.

Two other concerns involving the living will can be seen in the ICU. The first is when a patient who cannot respond has no living will. When this happens, the DPOA then has to guess which medical care the patient would want. So, it is important to have a plan in case the worst happens. The second concern is when a DPOA contradicts the patient's living will and pushes for unwanted medical care. Luckily, these situations can be avoided if the right DPOA is chosen and informed of the patient's wishes (page 137).

Provided below is a guide for a living will. Ideally, these medical scenarios are discussed early and often, before a decision is needed. Additionally, this should be revisited after any major life changes or loss of ability, especially during the hospitalization. The patient can get a better understanding of what effects the treatments have by discussing them with the ICU team. It is essential to focus on what the patient values in life, how the treatments affect daily life, and how long to pursue the treatments.

Living Will—Choosing your medical care now in case you cannot make decisions about it later.

- Situations (4 categories are listed here)
  - Incapacitated (brain injury, severe infection, etc)
    - Do you want:
      - Breathing tube (page 86)
      - Tracheostomy (page 42)
      - Tube feeding (page 34)
      - PEG tube (page 36)
      - Total parenteral nutrition (page 90)
      - Dialysis (page 75)
      - Blood transfusion (page 26)
      - Antibiotics
      - Surgery
    - Improvement in a certain amount of time?
    - Improvement to have a certain ability (being able to walk, communicate, etc)?
  - Emergency (heart stops [page 126] or breathing stops [page 86])

- ○ Do you want:
  - – Breathing tube
  - – Chest compressions
  - – Shock to restart your heart
  - – Medications to restart your heart
  - ○ Improvement in a certain amount of time?
  - ○ Improvement to have a certain ability (being able to walk, communicate, etc)?
- ● Approaching death or choosing to decline life support therapies
  - ○ Do you want:
    - – Medicine for pain, nausea, anxiety, shortness of breath?
    - – Certain people present?
    - – Music?
  - ○ Do you have religious or spiritual requests?
  - ○ Does it matter where you die (home or hospital)?
- ● After-death preferences
  - ○ Do you prefer burial, cremation, or donation to medical education or research?
  - ○ Do you want to be an organ donor? (page 133)
- ■ Make these choices known (the process depends on your state).
  - ● Make the living will official legally.
  - ● Consider uploading the document to an online registry so it can be easily accessed if needed.
  - ● Discuss with your DPOA and family.
  - ● Give copies to your doctors and bring one to the hospital.
  - ● See NavigatingTheICU.com for resources on how to get started.

Nurse's Note

- ■ You can be as general or specific as you want, but more detail will help the DPOA make the decision you would want.

- ■ For each therapy, you can accept, decline, or defer to the DPOA's judgment. If you defer to the DPOA, you can add comments. These could include a timeframe for recovery, or accepting the therapy only if you will probably recover abilities that allow for a life worth living.

- ■ Having a discussion with someone who experienced the therapy or a medical professional who understands what life is like for someone in these situations is important. They can explain how the medical care affects patients on a day-to-day basis. Researching this online is a good second option.

- ■ If this method is not working for you, please see the next section, Goal of Living Until Death, for another way to plan these decisions.

Goal of Living Until Death

How to Think About What Is Important

The goal of living until death is a way to think about what should be included in the living will. The idea loses abilities with age, yet many are still able to enjoy life. This is true until some point when too many abilities are lost to remain content.

The job here is to think of what is too important to lose and what can be sacrificed. This practice can include as many abilities and goals as needed. It can also include debilities that have to be avoided. Some of these may be simple choices, such as whether it is OK to need the ventilator to live. Others may be more difficult, like whether the ability to taste food is important. By choosing what makes a life worth living, the DPOA and medical team can aim the medical care to fulfill the patient's wishes.

It may be difficult to predict exactly what will make someone's life content. However, the patient needs to make this choice. Only the patient knows which abilities and debilities can be combined to create a desirable life. Only the patient knows which abilities and debilities can be combined to create a desirable life. The alternative is to let someone else guess which abilities could be lost and which debilities could be tolerated.

To come up with a list, think of abilities that are needed or situations that are unacceptable. With these choices, consider a timeframe around the decision. For instance, if a ventilator is needed for 1 month, would that be OK? Does this change if it is needed for 6 months or for life? Everything does not need an answer or direction. This should be revisited after major life changes, when any abilities are lost, and over the course of a hospitalization. Importantly, if a patient needs life support to survive an illness, but it will cost essential abilities or add unwanted debilities, comfort care should become the focus (page 152).

- What priorities and goals are needed in life?
  - Eating
  - Cooking
  - Walking
  - Exercise
  - Watching TV
  - Attending events
  - Being with someone
  - Being in remission

- Being at home
- Communicating with people
- Recognizing people
- _____
- _____

■ What situations would make life not worth living?
- Shortness of breath
- Fatigue
- Pain
- Not being able to control bowels or bladder
- Not being able to move the legs (paraplegia) or legs and arms (quadriplegia)
- Needing the ventilator (page 86)
- Needing to breathe through a hole in the windpipe (tracheostomy) (page 42)
- Needing to be fed through a hole into the stomach (PEG tube) (page 36)
- Needing a hole in abdomen to urinate or defecate (nephrostomy, colostomy)
- Needing dialysis multiple days per week (page 75)
- Needing help bathing, going to the bathroom, moving, or eating
- Full-time care in a rehabilitation facility (page 112)
- Full-time care from family
- Being your family's financial responsibility
- Unable to communicate
- Unable to recognize people
- Unable to make your own decisions
- _____
- _____

Nurse's Note

■ Having a discussion with someone who experienced the therapy or a medical professional who understands what life is like for someone in these situations is important. They can explain how the medical care affects patients on a day-to-day basis. Researching this online is a good second option.

■ The DPOA needs to know these choices, and they need to be outlined in your advance directives.

A Story of the Importance of Advance Care Planning

Brenda was a patient in the ICU. She was totally awake and aware of everything. She could see, hear, smell, taste, and feel. However, she could not lift a finger, scream for help, take a breath, or control her bowels. She could only move one part of her body, her eyes. This was her only way to communicate.

As I held a board with all 26 letters of the alphabet, I followed her eyes as they darted down, down, and left. Matching each eye movement with my finger, I moved from letter to letter, down, down, left. "P?" I guessed. She closed her eyes, confirming the first letter of what she was trying to tell me. She opened her eyes, and I reset my finger in the middle of the board. Up, up, left, left: A. Eyes closed. Down, down, right: I. Eyes closed. Down, left: N. I asked "pain?" before her eyes closed, trying to speed up the frustratingly slow process. She closed her eyes. "Where?" I responded. Right, left, down, up: L…E…G…S. For everything Brenda needed to say, this was the only way.

She tried to communicate her needs in the fewest letters possible. Mistakes occurred often, forcing us to start from the beginning. A board with Brenda's most common requests was made, but many things still needed to be spelled out with her eyes, letter by letter. Many requests were abandoned from frustration and exhaustion.

Brenda had Guillain-Barre syndrome, which causes paralysis. Everything was working normally except her ability to move. Thankfully, her eyes were spared. Brenda needed the breathing machine (ventilator) because she could not breathe on her own. This controlled her breathing through a hole in her windpipe (tracheostomy). She could not swallow, so we gave her liquid food through a tube into her stomach (PEG tube). The nurses had to reposition her so she did not develop any pressure injuries and bathe her after she soiled herself.

We spent many hours with Brenda, but mostly she lay in bed alone without any control. Only by looking in her eyes could you sense her terror. Anxiety was one of the words on her board.

By the end of the first month, Brenda became confused (delirious), and the medical team could no longer tell if she could make her own decisions (capacity). By law, the decisions about her medical care were then transferred to her closest next of kin, her estranged sister (DPOA). When we called her sister, she was surprised to hear of her new responsibilities. They had not spoken in years. At this point, Brenda had no control over what was going to happen to her.

Her sister thought that Brenda's goal was to get healthy (goals of care), so the medical team directed their therapy to make this happen. After another month of paralysis, anxiety, and delirium, the disorder gave way, and she slowly regained her abilities.

Because of all the time spent in bed, Brenda was so weak she could not lift her hands off of the bed (post-intensive care syndrome). She was transferred to a special facility where she spent months regaining her strength and learning how to walk again (rehabilitation). She had to learn how to speak, this time using a speaking valve with her tracheostomy. Eventually, Brenda did get better and was able to return home.

I share Brenda's story for a few reasons. The first is to show what life can be like with advanced medical care. For many people, Brenda's worst experiences are their daily lives. When thinking about your own goals of care, it can be helpful to know how the medical care can affect your daily life. Some people are content with these changes, while others are not. Only you can decide for yourself.

The second reason is to emphasize the importance of a time-frame. Some people want to pursue all medical options no matter how long it takes, while others cannot bear the idea of being on life support indefinitely. For Brenda, it turns out that she never wanted to experience that time of incapacitation. She was OK giving the medical care a chance for the first month. But she then could not change her mind after she lost her capacity. She did not have a living will or DPOA who knew her wishes, so the decision to continue therapy was made for her. When recovered, Brenda admitted that she wished nature would have taken its course after the first month rather than live through the traumatic experience. She was fortunate her illness did not continue much longer. Some people are trapped in her situation for their entire lives. They missed the opportunity to tell their DPOA how long they were willing to try to reach their goals of care.

The third reason is to show the importance of picking the right DPOA and communicating your wishes for a life worth living. Brenda's preference for her medical care was given to her sister, who was unfamiliar with Brenda's wishes. Her sister thought that she was doing the right thing, especially because Brenda survived. However, the medical care provided should have been what

Brenda desired. In this case, she would have rather peacefully died than live through that experience. Even though her DPOA thought it was the right decision and she survived, it was the wrong decision for Brenda. Therefore, you must be sure you know who your DPOA is and confirm that they can make tough decisions to support the life and death you want. Many times, the family chooses the most aggressive care with the hope that the patient will recover. Truly, only by discussing these situations with your DPOA will they know your goals of living and be able to protect your medical future.

Physician Orders for Life-Sustaining Treatment (POLST or Medical OLST)

If the Patient is Likely to Get Seriously Ill Within one Year

In the event the provider believes the patient may require critical medical decisions to be made within one year, a physician orders for life-sustaining treatment (POLST) form may be necessary. Directly personalized for the patient, a POLST outlines what orders all medical personnel will follow for the patient. Each state has different rules regarding this type of document, and the medical provider can explain the specifics. Even with a POLST, it is still important to communicate with a trustworthy DPOA who will make decisions according to the patient's requests.

Nurse's Note

- The name may be different depending on your state.
- Discuss with the provider if this advance directive interests you. There may be a different form in your state that would best serve your loved one.

Helpful Online Resources to Organize Thoughts

There are many different advance directives, and they can change depending on your state. To make this process easier, this book includes a few resources below that are helpful, and the links are available at NavigatingTheICU.com. As always, the ICU staff are available for any assistance, advice, or conversation.

The American Bar Association has helpful documents for advance care planning. They discuss how to plan for what may come, how to choose a DPOA, and helpful tips for the DPOA.

MyRegistry provides the ability to create a living will and choose a DPOA. Advance directives can also be uploaded. They can be saved online to be shared with anyone or accessed by healthcare providers.

The National Hospice and Palliative Care Organization has many resources to explain advance care planning and create advance directives.

Nurse's Note

- You can and should reassess these documents. Your preferences may change over time.
- These documents can help to reduce the burden felt by your DPOA when a decision needs to be made.
- Ask your medical team if any other advance directives are needed for you or your loved one.
- Be sure to double-check your state's rules.

If the Patient Cannot Respond, and the Family Does Not Know Their Wishes

Teaming With the ICU Staff to Make Sure the Patient's Care Is the Right Care

Many families have not had a conversation with their loved one about their medical preferences. This is OK. This is very common. When this occurs, reviewing the patient's life and comparing it with their probable recovery can help guide decisions. This typically happens in a goals of care meeting.

A goals of care meeting is when the ICU team and family gather to discuss the best path forward for the patient. This can be referred to as a family meeting. Usually, this meeting is called because the patient's illness is severe, and decisions are needed about the direction of their treatment.

The meeting begins by introducing everyone. The ICU team may ask what the family knows about the patient's current illness. Then, the ICU team may summarize what has happened with the patient so far. They may also be interested in what the patient was like before the illness. For instance, the ICU team may ask about the patient's life story, what they enjoy doing, and what they value in life. The ICU team wants to understand their values, learn about their preferences, and try to grasp what made life worth living for the patient. The family helps the ICU team see if the current medical care is right for the patient.

The ICU team may also discuss what the usual recovery is like for patients in this situation. The amount of recovery needed, where it takes place, and for how long can give the family an idea of what the patient's future looks like. If this future is not right for the patient, the ICU team and family work together to develop a plan that best serves the patient.

Nurse's Note

- Answers for the patient's future may not be clear. All that the family and ICU team can do is use their experience and knowledge to help guide this conversation.

- It may be helpful to imagine what your loved one would say if they could wake up for only 10 minutes, see everything that is happening to them, and understand what the future probably looks like.

- It may help to bring other family and friends for support. They can contribute, listen, and help remember (or write down) details when thinking about the meeting later.

- It may be possible to have this meeting over the phone or video call, or to include important people over the phone or video call.

- Please see the sections, Living Will (page 139) and Goal of Living Until Death (page 142) for ideas of what would make life worth living for your loved one.

15

Important Topics When Discussing the End of the Patient's Life

This chapter focuses on some of the options available when the current medical care may not accomplish the patient's goals of care. First, different directions of care that may be pursued are defined. Then, options are presented for those who need more time to make a decision. Finally, how the medical team and family join to comfort the patient in their last moments is explained.

Palliative care serves to reduce suffering. Sometimes confused with hospice, palliative care is provided to all patients, including those who are not near the end of life. In fact, all medical care has an element of palliative care within it. When a patient recovers from an operation, pain medicine, symptom management, and helping the person cope with any bodily changes are all considered palliative.

Some hospitals have a palliative care team that specializes in providing palliative care to those with serious illnesses. This team works with the ICU team. Made up of providers, nurses, and other medical staff, they focus on what is reducing the patient's ability to enjoy life. This team tries to improve the patient's quality of life by relieving physical and emotional discomfort. They can also assist in helping to align the medical care with the patient's goals of care. Sometimes, this may mean shifting the focus to comfort care (page 152). Importantly, palliative care can occur at the same time medical care tries to cure a patient.

Nurse's Note

■ The sooner palliative care occurs, the better. Patients and families benefit from this extra layer of support, especially when it is started early in the illness.

■ If available at your hospital, you may have to request the palliative care team for them to come see you.

■ A palliative care team consultation may be paid for by your insurance. You can always double-check with the medical team.

Hospice care is used when curing the illness is not the patient's focus. It includes palliative care but is specifically used in end-of-life situations. If a provider determines that a patient has less than 6 months to live, they can recommend hospice care.

Typically, the medical interventions to cure the illness are stopped, but measures are still taken to treat physical and emotional discomfort. For instance, pain, nausea, and anxiety medication can be given to allow patients more quality time doing what they want. This can take place at home or in a healthcare facility.

In no way is hospice "giving up." It is a shift in focus toward spending less time trying to be cured and spending more time on what matters for the patient. When time is limited, this different focus is important for some patients. This can improve their satisfaction with life. For instance, some feel that it is more valuable to spend their remaining time at home with family rather than at the hospital receiving medical care.

A hospice team helps the patient with their goals of care. This team can include a provider, nurse, social worker, and spiritual services. Other resources may be available, such as physical therapy, occupational therapy, a speech-language pathologist, and medical equipment. The hospice team can also support the family. They may suggest respite care (someone who gives the family caregiver a break), grieving support, and other resources that are commonly appreciated.

Nurse's Note

■ The cost may be covered by insurance, but you can always ask to double-check.

■ To see the quality of care a hospice provides, you can ask how they measure their care and to see the data. You may be able to compare this to other hospice facilities.

Comfort care is a term used in the ICU when further treatment no longer matches the patient's goals of care. This is the decision to stop the patient's life-supporting medical therapy. This medical care is keeping the patient alive, but it also may be prolonging their suffering. The patient's life-preserving therapies—such as medications to support blood pressure and the breathing tube—are traded for measures aimed at relieving distress. The decision for comfort care is made by the patient with capacity or the durable power of attorney. If the patient does not die quickly, they can be transferred to hospice. The Comfort Care section covers this process in more detail (page 152).

If More Time Is Needed to Decide About the Right Path for the Patient

Many people are overwhelmed or unsure when deciding if end-of-life options are right for their loved one. Usually, important questions cannot be given clear answers. Therefore, concerned family members feel as if they do not have enough information to make the decision between continuing treatment and focusing on comfort care (page 152).

For one thing, it is OK if more time is needed. The family should tell this to the medical team. Then, a plan can be made for the family to have a reasonable amount of time to make sure they can make the best decision. Decisions do not need to be rushed, but they do need to be made.

Some other options in these moments are time-limited trials and to not escalate treatment. A time-limited trial involves giving the patient a certain amount of time to respond to treatments. If there are signs of recovery within that time, the treatments can continue. If there are no signs of recovery within that time, the family and medical team can approach comfort care knowing they gave the treatments and patient a chance. A second option is to not escalate treatment. This means that the current aggressive medical care is continued. However, no additional medical treatments to prolong life will be added, even if the patient's health worsens. If the patient's heart stops, the medical team will not try to restart it. Those who do not want to remove life-supporting therapy may prefer this. However, continuing medical treatment prevents the ICU team from ensuring that the patient is as comfortable as possible. Importantly, these choices should still serve the patient's goals of care.

If families think the situation is not being explored fairly, the ethics committee can be asked for an opinion. They are separate from the patient's ICU team. This group has experience negotiating difficult situations, and they can help to resolve issues between those who disagree.

Whenever a serious decision needs to be made, a second opinion can be requested to explore all of the options. This request can be brought to the medical team. Please see the Second Opinion section for more details (page 125).

The decision to continue aggressive care needs to include a meeting with the medical team. It is essential to discuss how these treatments are going to affect the patient's daily life. Furthermore, it is important to know where these treatments will take place (ICU, skilled nursing facility, home, etc, page 112) and who will be providing care in those settings. The financial and time commitments also have to be realized. The last thing anyone wants is to be unable to care for their loved one because the commitments necessary were not understood.

Comfort Care: A Focus on Patient Comfort as Death Nears

The goal of <u>comfort care</u> is to soothe the patient's mind and body as the medical care prolonging their life and the illness is stopped. This decision is made when continuing the medical therapy will not help the patient live their desired life.

Focusing on comfort is not killing the patient. Extraordinary medical care is the only reason this very sick patient is still alive. Without this support, death would have already occurred. This change of focus allows the patient to rest in comfort without prolonging the pains of their illness. This decision eases the patient from their struggle and grants a natural, peaceful death.

The comfort care process is explained below. There are questions the family usually asks. Some of these are: how long until the patient passes, will the patient feel anything, does the family stay in the room for the entire process, and what happens after? The answer to each question depends on the patient, but the typical responses are mentioned here. Of course, the entire medical team is available if anything is needed.

Each ICU has different ways to help the family honor and comfort their loved one in these moments. Some examples include printing their heartbeat, seen on the monitor, or taking a print of their hands. Some families like to bring the patient their favorite things, such as a blanket, stuffed animal, or pictures. It may also be comforting to give the patient a shave, moisten their mouth, play their favorite music, cool their forehead with a wet washcloth, or paint their nails. Some of the patient's favorite simple pleasures may be allowed during this time. A chaplain, spiritual services, and social worker can be requested as well.

Nurse's Note

- If any of these interest you, please check with the nurse to see if they are possible.
- You can ask the ICU staff if they have other ideas or resources for these moments.

The organ donation organization may make contact to discuss donation. If there is interest in organ donation and no communication has been made, please let the nurse know.

When the decision is made to transition to comfort care, only medications that make the patient comfortable are given. A combination of medications is used. Opioids, such as morphine, reduce pain and the feeling of not being able to get enough air, known as air hunger. Benzodiazepines, such as midazolam, reduce anxiety. An anticholinergic, glycopyrrolate, reduces saliva production to prevent coughing. Importantly, the patient is not aware of any discomfort during this time.

Other medical equipment and procedures prolonging life may be stopped. A common life-supporting therapy to remove is the breathing tube. This occurs after the family and medical team are ready. Although it is not painful, some feel that they do not want to watch. It involves suctioning saliva out of the mouth, deflating the cuff holding the tube in position, and pulling it out. Usually, oxygen is not provided because it is considered a life-supporting therapy.

After these therapies are stopped, the ICU team continues to comfort the patient in all possible ways. The staff stops unnecessary medical care, tries to create a soothing environment, and can give more medications, if needed. The patient may sound like they are breathing through saliva. Sometimes referred to as a death rattle, it is more upsetting to the family than the patient. Unfortunately, it can be hard to suction out, and trying to remove it can cause discomfort. Of course, the family is welcome to ask the nurse to try this or other things to comfort the patient.

Family can hold the patient's hand, play their favorite music, talk to the patient, or do whatever feels natural. The time until death depends on the patient's illness, and the medical team can provide guidance.

After passing, the family is given time to spend with the patient. Unfortunately, ICU beds are needed at all hours, and rooms have to be prepared for another sick patient. The nurse can give an estimate for how much time can be spent in the room. After the family leaves, the ICU staff sends the patient to the morgue. After-death arrangements are usually made with the funeral home. The nurse will cover these details with the family.

Nurse's Note

- You may feel that you do not want to be present as the patient passes. This is equally OK as being at the bedside. Rest assured, your loved one is comfortable and is not dying alone.

- If you cannot make it to the bedside, joining the patient by video call may be an option. You can ask the nurse if this is possible.

- The health of your mind, body, and emotions are important to your healing. Please see Chapter 11 (page 105) as you recover from this time.

- The ICU may have a bereavement packet that goes over the decisions that need to be made after the death of a loved one. It can be hard to process anything in these moments, and this packet can simplify things. If one is not available, you can ask the team to write down what needs to be done and who to contact with questions.

Glossary

Pronunciations courtesy of Stedman's Online.

Acute (ă-kyūt′) – An issue that is new, progresses quickly, or is severe.

"We think this is an acute illness because you have never experienced anything that made you feel this badly before."

Acute on Chronic (ă-kyūt′, kron′ik) – A sudden worsening of a patient's existing disease.

"Her new lung infection is making her already scarred lungs worse, so this is an acute on chronic illness."

Alert and Oriented (A and O) (ə′lərt, ′ôrē,ən-ted) – Way to assess brain function by asking the patient if they know their name, the date, where they are, and why they are there.

"He is A and O times two, he only knows his name and the date."

Anesthesia (an′es-thē′zē-ă) – The medicine or person providing comfort during a procedure.

"The anesthetic is preventing the patient from feeling pain."

Anoxia (an-ok′sē-ă) – No oxygen in the body.

"If he had not received oxygen, the anoxia would have damaged his brain."

Artery (ahŕtĕr-ē) – Blood vessels that carry oxygenated blood from the heart to the organs.

"We can see how much oxygen is in the body with a sample of the arterial blood."

Aspirate (as′pi-rāt) – To inhale something into the lungs, usually food or liquid.

"I wonder if he aspirated because he started having trouble breathing right after dinner."

Baseline (bās′līn) – A patient's normal.

"He has low blood pressure at baseline and feels fine."

Bedrest (bed rest) – Staying in bed to help with recovery.

"The patient is on bedrest until we can increase his blood pressure."

Blood Clot (blŭd klot) – A ball of blood cells that stick together and can clog blood vessels.

"We prevent blood clots from forming with medicine and encouraging getting out of bed."

Bolus (bō′lŭs) – Giving a large amount of something over a short period of time.

"Because she is in so much pain, we are going to give her a bolus of pain medicine."

Bradycardia (brad′ē-kahr′dē-ă) – Slow heart rate. Usually, lower than 60.

"As long as she feels OK, we are not worried about her bradycardia."

Bradypnea (brad′ip-nē′ă) – Slow breathing rate.

"We may have to help her breathe faster if she continues to be this bradypneic."

Cannula (kan′yū-lă) – A tube.

"Oxygen is travelling through the nasal cannula into her nose."

Cardiac (kahr′dē-ak) – Referring to the heart.

"His heart appears to be working great after the medications to support his cardiac function."

Catheter (kath′ĕ-tĕr) – A tube.

"Medicine is given through her IV catheter into her bloodstream."

Cerebral (sə-′rē-brəl) – Referring to the brain.

"I am not worried about any cerebral damage because she is acting normally."

Chronic (kron′ik) – An issue that is persistent or reoccurs.

"Tell me what usually helps with your chronic back pain that you have had for years."

Clot (klot) – A ball of blood cells that stick together and can clog blood vessels.

"We worry that if you do not get out of bed, a clot can form in your legs."

Compensate (kom′pĕn-sāt) – The body's temporary ability to adjust to problems.

"He is compensating for his low oxygen levels by taking many deep and rapid breaths."

Competence (kom′pĕ-tĕns) – The patient's ability to make decisions that align with their goals of care.

"She is competent because she can understand the different options and make a logical choice."

Complication (kom′pli-kā′shŭn) – An unintended, negative effect of medical treatment.

"The blood clot he developed was a serious complication from the medicine."

Constrict (kən′strikt) – To narrow or tighten up.

"An allergic reaction constricts the throat and can make it hard to breathe."

Contrast (kon′trast) – Medicine that allows body structures and fluids to be seen on imaging.

"The CT with contrast shows a blocked blood vessel in the brain."

Critical (krit′ĭ-kăl) – When a patient's health is worsening or may worsen quickly.

"She is still in critical condition, so we will keep a close eye on her in case she gets worse."

CT Scan (Computed Tomography (kŏm-pyū′tĕd tŏ-mog′ră-fē), Cat Scan) – An O-shaped machine that takes many X-rays to get a very detailed look of the inside of the patient's body.

"To see if she had a brain injury, we are taking her for a CT scan of her brain."

Desaturate/Desat (dē-sat′yū-rāt/ dē-sat) – When a patient has a sudden decrease in their oxygen levels.

"She desatted when she stood up, so I gave her more oxygen."

Diagnosis (dī-ăg-nō′sis) – Identifying the illness or problem.

"Based on the symptoms and tests, the patient's diagnosis is pneumonia."

Diastolic Blood Pressure (dī′ă-stol′ik blŭd presh′ŭr) – Blood pressure when the heart is relaxed between beats.

"Her diastolic blood pressure is probably higher because of her stress."

Dilate (dī′lāt) – To widen or open up.

"Some medications dilate the blood vessels to allow more blood into the area."

Discharge (dis′chahrj) – (1) Leaving the hospital.

"Because you're getting discharged home within the week, mention any questions you have about life after the hospital."

(2) Fluid leaking from an area

"Because the IV site is red and there is discharge coming from it, I am worried it might be infected."

Dressing (dres′ing) – Protective cover.

"The central line dressing is falling off, so I am going to change it."

Drip (drip) – Fluid or medication given continuously through an IV.

"We are starting a drip to make sure her blood pressure is OK."

DVT (Deep Vein Thrombosis (dēp vān throm-bō′sis)) – A blood clot in a vein, usually in the legs.

"The swelling and pain in only one of her legs was a warning sign of a DVT."

Dye (dī) – Medicine that allows body structures and fluids to be seen on imaging.

"The head CT will use dye to see where the brain injury is."

Dyspnea (disp-nē′ă) – When a patient is having trouble breathing.

"You can tell she is dyspneic because she is working so hard to breathe and looks uncomfortable."

Echo (Echocardiogram (ek′ō-kahr′dē-ō-gram)) – A test that uses sound waves to measure the size of the different parts of the heart and how well they are working.

"Every patient with this heart problem receives an echo."

EKG/ECG (Electrocardiogram (ĕ-lek′trō-kahr′dē-ō-gram)) – A test that measures the electrical signal of the heart to tell how well it is beating.

"Because her EKG looks different, we will take some labs to see how her heart is working."

End-Tidal CO_2 (end-tī′dăl c. o. 2) – The amount of carbon dioxide exhaled. Usually, normal is 35-45.

"Her end-tidal CO_2 is 40, meaning she is breathing normally."

Enteral Nutrition (en′tĕr-ăl nū-trish′ŭn) – Liquid nutrition that is given through a tube into the stomach or intestines.

"Because he cannot eat enough, we will give him extra calories with enteral nutrition."

Failure (fāl′yŭr) When a body function stops working, which disrupts the entire body's ability to work normally.

"His lung failure is causing him to not breathe in enough oxygen."

Fluid (flū′ld) – Water mixed with electrolytes that are usually given through an IV for hydration.

"We are giving her fluids to replace all that she has lost from vomiting and diarrhea."

Follow-up (fol′ō-ŭp) – Meeting with medical personnel at a later time to discuss an issue.

"Let's follow-up in a week to make sure you are still feeling OK."

GI (Gastrointestinal (gas′trō-in-tes′ti-năl)) – Referring to the digestive system made up the mouth, esophagus, stomach, small intestine, large intestine, and anus.

"It is normal for his GI tract to be slow following surgery."

Glucose (glū′kōs) – Blood sugar.

"We test his blood sugar every six hours to make sure his glucose levels are normal."

Heart Rate (hahrt rāt) – The number of heartbeats per minute. Usually, 60-100 is normal.

"If you feel fine, a heart rate lower than 60 is OK."

Hepatic (hĕ-pat′ik) – Referring to the liver.

"Judging from the labs that measure liver function, he has had some hepatic damage."

Hypercarbia (hī′pĕr-kahr′bē-ă) – Buildup of carbon dioxide in the blood. Usually, higher than 45.

"This will make him breathe faster so he is not as hypercarbic."

Hypertension (hī′pĕr-ten′shŭn) – High blood pressure. This number depends on the ICU patient.

"Patients with that level of hypertension usually have to take medication to lower their blood pressure."

Hypoglycemia (hī′pō-glī-sē′mē-ă) – Low blood sugar, usually lower than 70.

"To prevent hypoglycemia, we will give him some fluids with sugar."

Hypotension (hī′pō-ten′shŭn) – Low blood pressure, usually lower than a MAP of 65 or systolic blood pressure of 90.

"She is hypotensive, so we are giving her medicine to bring up her blood pressure."

Hypothermia (hī′pō-thĕr′mē-ă) – Low body temperature, usually lower than 95°F.

"We are using blankets to warm her because she arrived hypothermic."

Hypoxia (hī-pok′sē-ă) – Low oxygen levels in the body.

"His toes are blue because he is hypoxic."

Incentive Spirometer (in-sen′tiv spr·aa· muh·tr) – A tool to help strengthen the lungs.

"If you use the incentive spirometer every hour, you will probably get out of the ICU sooner."

Incontinent (in-kon′ti-nĕnt) – Unable to control bladder and/or bowels.

"Because she is incontinent, we have to clean her skin often."

Infusion (in-fyū′zhŭn) – Fluid, medication, or blood given through an IV.

"The continuous IV fluid infusion will continue for the next few days."

Insertion Site (in-sĕr′shŭn sīt) – Where the medical device enters the body.

"The central line insertion site looks red, so I think it may have to be removed."

Intervention (in′tĕr-ven′shŭn) – Acting to change a patient's condition.

"The intervention to return blood flow to his heart saved his life."

Intravenous (in′tră-vē′nŭs) – Into a vein.

"The pain medicine is being given intravenously through her IV."

Invasive (in-vā′siv) – A therapy that is inserted into the body.

"The procedure will be invasive because we have to make a small hole in your skin."

Isolation (ī′sŏ-lā′shŭn) – Using protective gear and a protective room to prevent spreading an infection from a patient or to a patient.

"Because his cough can spread the virus, he is in isolation."

IV Nutrition (i.v. nū-trish'ŭn) – Nutrition given through an IV.

"To help her regain strength while she cannot eat, she will receive IV nutrition for a few weeks."

Level of Consciousness (lev'ĕl, kon'shŭs-nĕs) – How the patient is thinking and acting.

"We are worried about his brain because his level of consciousness changed."

Life Support (līf sŭp-ōrt') – Any medical therapy that supports or replaces a failing organ.

"The medication supporting his heart is the only life support he is on right now."

Mean Arterial Pressure (MAP) (mēn ahr-tēr'ē-ăl presh'ŭr) – The average blood pressure in the arteries. Usually, higher than 65 is OK.

"If the MAP is less than 65 we give more medicine to raise the blood pressure."

Melena (mĕ-lē'nă) – Stool that contains blood, making it dark and tarry.

"We think there is a bleed somewhere in the upper GI tract because of the melena."

Mental Status/Mentation (men'tăl stat'ŭs/men-tā'shŭn) – How the patient is thinking and acting.

"Because his mental status changed, we are worried he may have a brain injury."

Mobilize (mō'bi-līz) – Exercising by working out in the bed or getting out of the bed.

"Try to mobilize to the chair today so you can build up your strength."

Monitor (mon'i-tŏr) – The device that shows the patient's vital signs.

"He is connected to the monitor at all times, so we will be able to see if his heart rate changes."

MRI (Magnetic Resonance Imaging) (mag-net'ik rez'ŏ-năns im'ăj-ing) – An O-shaped machine that takes the most detailed images of the inside of the patient's body.

"The brain MRI will be able to show exactly where the brain injury is."

Normal Sinus Rhythm (nōr'măl sī'nŭs ri-thəm) – A normal heartbeat, usually 60-100 times per minute.

"She has been in normal sinus rhythm throughout her hospital stay."

OR (Operating Room) (op'ĕr-āt-ing rūm) – Where surgeries take place.

"He will be in the OR for a couple of hours, so this is a good time to get lunch."

Ostomy (os'tŏ-mē) – A surgically created opening to remove feces or urine.

"The ostomy is needed after the large intestine infection."

Oxygen Saturation (ok-si'jĕn sach'ŭr-ā'shŭn) – The percentage of oxygen in the blood. Usually, higher than 92 is OK.

"Because lower oxygen levels are normal for her, we are OK with oxygen saturations higher than 90."

Patient Safety Attendant (pā'shĕnt sāf'tē ə'tendənt) – A medical professional who watches a patient to make sure they are safe.

"The patient safety attendant will watch your father at night to make sure he does not try to get out of bed and fall."

Plan of Care (plan, kār) – The medical plan for the patient's illness.

"The plan of care is to treat the infection with antibiotics while monitoring the patient for any complications."

PO (p.o.) – Swallowing medications, food, or liquid.

"Be careful with anything PO because we're not sure if he can safely swallow."

Perfusion (pĕr-fyū′zhŭn) – Blood flow to an area.

"His toes are cold because of the weak perfusion to his feet."

Pressor (pres′ŏr) – A medication that increases blood pressure.

"She will need pressors to bring her blood pressure up to a healthy level."

Prognosis (prog-nō′sis) – Predicting the course of the illness or problem.

"The prognosis is poor because the patient is very sick."

Provider (prō-vī′dĕr) – A doctor, nurse practitioner, or physician assistant who diagnoses an illness and prescribes treatments for the patient.

"The provider ordered the medicine and asked the nurse to administer it."

Pulmonary (pul′mŏ-nār-ē) – Referring to the lungs.

"I think he is breathing better today, which shows that his pulmonary issues are improving."

Referred Pain (rĕ-fĕrd′ pān) – Pain that is felt somewhere besides the location of the injury.

"A chest tube usually causes referred pain in the shoulder."

Rehabilitation/Rehab (rē′hă-bil′i-tā′shŭn/rē′hăb) – Working to recover abilities.

"After the fall, the patient will need rehab with physical therapy to walk safely again."

Renal (rē′năl) – Referring to the kidneys.

"After the infection reached her kidneys, she appeared to have renal damage."

Respiratory Distress (res′pir-ă-tōr-ē dis-tres′) – When a patient is having trouble breathing.

"If his respiratory distress gets worse, we may have to insert the breathing tube."

Respiratory Rate (res′pir-ă-tōr-ē rāt) – The number of breaths per minute. Usually, 12-20 is normal.

"It is normal to have a respiratory rate lower than 12 when sleeping."

Sats (sats) – The percentage of oxygen in the blood. Usually, higher than 92 is considered OK.

"Her sats improved after we gave her more oxygen."

Secretion (sĕ-krē′shŭn) – Saliva and phlegm in the mouth, throat, and lungs.

"The ventilator is alarming because her secretions are causing her to cough."

Sepsis (sep′sis) – When an infection causes the body to function poorly.

"She looks septic, so we are going to give her antibiotics and closely monitor her."

Shock (shok) – When the body's tissues do not receive oxygen.

"Because the heart cannot pump blood well after the heart attack, the patient is in shock."

Sitter (sit-er) – A medical professional who watches a patient to make sure they are safe.

"The sitter will watch your father at night to make sure he does not try to get out of bed and fall."

Somnolent (som′nō-lĕnt) – Sleepy.

"I am worried he will choke on his food because he is somnolent."

Sputum (spyū′tŭm) – Saliva and phlegm in the mouth, throat, and lungs.

"Coughing up the sputum will help her breathe easier."

Stable (stā′bĕl) – When a patient's health has only a small risk of suddenly worsening.

"Because he is so stable, I do not have to monitor him."

Stoma (stō′mă) – A hole or opening created in the body to help with its functioning.

"A surgically created stoma in your trachea will help you breathe easier."

Symptom (sĭmp′tŏm) – A clue the patient's body gives about an illness or a problem.

"Judging from your symptoms, we think you may have an infection."

Systolic Blood Pressure (sis-tol′ik blŭd presh′ŭr) – Blood pressure when the heart beats/squeezes.

"Her systolic blood pressure is too high, so we will have to lower it with medicine."

Tachycardia (tak′i-kahr′dē-ă) – Fast heart rate, usually higher than 100.

"It is common for a fever to cause tachycardia."

Tachypnea (tak′ip-nē′ă) – Fast breathing rate, usually higher than 20.

"His anxiety is causing him to be so tachypneic."

Tissue (tish′ū) – Different parts of the body that make up the organs.

"The tissues need oxygen or else the organs may be hurt."

Titrate (tī′trāt) – To adjust the amount of a therapy.

"The nurse titrates the amount of oxygen until the patient feels comfortable."

Total Parenteral Nutrition (TPN) (tō′tăl pă-ren′tĕr-ăl nū-trish′ŭn) – Nutrition given through an IV.

"She will get TPN for a week while her intestines heal from surgery."

Tube Feed (tūb fēd) – Liquid nutrition that is given through a tube into the stomach or intestines.

"While she has the breathing tube, she will be fed with tube feeds."

Unstable (ŭn-stā′bĕl) – When a patient's health is worsening or may worsen quickly.

"We have to be prepared for anything because this patient is so unstable."

Vasodilator (vā′sō-dī′lā-tŏr) – A medication that decreases blood pressure.

"She will need vasodilators to bring her blood pressure down to a healthy level."

Vasopressor (vā′sō-pres′ŏr) – A medication that increases blood pressure.

"She will need vasopressors to bring her blood pressure up to a healthy level."

Vein (vān) – A blood vessel that carries blood back to the heart after delivering oxygen to the organs.

"All IVs are inserted into veins, and that is where the medication flows."

Wean (wēn) – To reduce the amount of a therapy.

"The nurse will wean the patient off of the sedation medication to wake him up."

X-ray (′eks-, rā) – The most common way to get an image of the inside of the patient's body.

"Compared to yesterday's chest X-ray, today's chest X-ray shows that the lung infection is improving."

Appendices

APPENDIX 1 Helpful Tool for Organizing Patient Details or to Use During Rounds

Use this to organize the many details about the patient and healthcare team. This can be used to keep track of past events, present concerns, and future plans. Each prompt may not be needed, and other important issues can be added. Also, please write at least one option for "What am I doing for self-care today?"

Date: _____ ICU Day #: _____

The patient's goals of care are (confirm with medical team):

Who is the medical team?

ICU Personnel	Name	Caring for Patient Until When?
Attending		
Resident/NP/PA		
Day Nurse		
Night Nurse		

Current issues (ask the ICU team for a list):

Plan for the day for each issue:

What needs to be followed up later and when is it scheduled?
    Schedule time for updates, visiting, video call?
    Labs/Tests/Procedures/Surgery?

Goals of the day:
    Spontaneous Awakening Trial?
    Spontaneous Breathing Trial?
    Physical/Occupational/Speech Therapy?
    Prevent Post-Intensive Care Syndrome
    Exercise/Get out of bed

Questions for the team:

Plans for discharge:
    Social worker/Case manager contacted about plans for after hospital?
    Anticipated date to leave ICU _____ and hospital _____?

What am I doing for self-care for today?

Date: _____ ICU Day #: _____

The patient's goals of care are (confirm with medical team):

Who is the medical team?

ICU Personnel	Name	Caring for Patient Until When?
Attending		
Resident/NP/PA		
Day Nurse		
Night Nurse		

Current issues (ask the ICU team for a list):

Plan for the day for each issue:

What needs to be followed up later and when is it scheduled?
Schedule time for updates, visiting, video call?
Labs/Tests/Procedures/Surgery?

Goals of the day:
Spontaneous Awakening Trial?
Spontaneous Breathing Trial?
Physical therapist/occupational therapist/speech-language pathologist?
Prevent Post-Intensive Care Syndrome
Exercise/Get out of bed

Questions for the team:

Plans for discharge:
Social worker/Case manager contacted about plans for after hospital?
Anticipated date to leave ICU _____ and hospital _____?

What am I doing for self-care for today?

Date: _____ ICU Day #: _____

The patient's goals of care are (confirm with medical team):

Who is the medical team?

ICU Personnel	Name	Caring for Patient Until When?
Attending		
Resident/NP/PA		
Day Nurse		
Night Nurse		

Current issues (ask the ICU team for a list):

Plan for the day for each issue:

What needs to be followed up later and when is it scheduled?
 Schedule time for updates, visiting, video call?
 Labs/Tests/Procedures/Surgery?

Goals of the day:
 Spontaneous Awakening Trial?
 Spontaneous Breathing Trial?
 Physical/Occupational/Speech Therapy?
 Prevent Post-Intensive Care Syndrome
 Exercise/Get out of bed

Questions for the team:

Plans for discharge:
 Social worker/Case manager contacted about plans for after hospital?
 Anticipated date to leave ICU _____ and hospital _____?

What am I doing for self-care for today?

Date: _____ ICU Day #: _____

The patient's goals of care are (confirm with medical team):

Who is the medical team?

ICU Personnel	Name	Caring for Patient Until When?
Attending		
Resident/NP/PA		
Day Nurse		
Night Nurse		

Current issues (ask the ICU team for a list):

Plan for the day for each issue:

What needs to be followed up later and when is it scheduled?
　Schedule time for updates, visiting, video call?
　Labs/Tests/Procedures/Surgery?

Goals of the day:
　Spontaneous Awakening Trial?
　Spontaneous Breathing Trial?
　Physical therapist/occupational therapist/speech-language pathologist?
　Prevent Post-Intensive Care Syndrome
　Exercise/Get out of bed

Questions for the team:

Plans for discharge:
　Social worker/Case manager contacted about plans for after hospital?
　Anticipated date to leave ICU _____ and hospital _____?

What am I doing for self-care for today?

Date: _____ ICU Day #: _____

The patient's goals of care are (confirm with medical team):

Who is the medical team?

ICU Personnel	Name	Caring for Patient Until When?
Attending		
Resident/NP/PA		
Day Nurse		
Night Nurse		

Current issues (ask the ICU team for a list):

Plan for the day for each issue:

What needs to be followed up later and when is it scheduled?
    Schedule time for updates, visiting, video call?
    Labs/Tests/Procedures/Surgery?

Goals of the day:
    Spontaneous Awakening Trial?
    Spontaneous Breathing Trial?
    Physical/Occupational/Speech Therapy?
    Prevent Post-Intensive Care Syndrome
    Exercise/Get out of bed

Questions for the team:

Plans for discharge:
    Social worker/Case manager contacted about plans for after hospital?
    Anticipated date to leave ICU _____ and hospital _____?

What am I doing for self-care for today?

Date: _____ ICU Day #: _____

The patient's goals of care are (confirm with medical team):

Who is the medical team?

ICU Personnel	Name	Caring for Patient Until When?
Attending		
Resident/NP/PA		
Day Nurse		
Night Nurse		

Current issues (ask the ICU team for a list):

Plan for the day for each issue:

What needs to be followed up later and when is it scheduled?
  Schedule time for updates, visiting, video call?
  Labs/Tests/Procedures/Surgery?

Goals of the day:
  Spontaneous Awakening Trial?
  Spontaneous Breathing Trial?
  Physical therapist/occupational therapist/speech-language pathologist?
  Prevent Post-Intensive Care Syndrome
  Exercise/Get out of bed

Questions for the team:

Plans for discharge:
  Social worker/Case manager contacted about plans for after hospital?
  Anticipated date to leave ICU _____ and hospital _____?

What am I doing for self-care for today?

Date: _____ ICU Day #: _____

The patient's goals of care are (confirm with medical team):

Who is the medical team?

ICU Personnel	Name	Caring for Patient Until When?
Attending		
Resident/NP/PA		
Day Nurse		
Night Nurse		

Current issues (ask the ICU team for a list):

Plan for the day for each issue:

What needs to be followed up later and when is it scheduled?
Schedule time for updates, visiting, video call?
Labs/Tests/Procedures/Surgery?

Goals of the day:
Spontaneous Awakening Trial?
Spontaneous Breathing Trial?
Physical/Occupational/Speech Therapy?
Prevent Post-Intensive Care Syndrome
Exercise/Get out of bed

Questions for the team:

Plans for discharge:
Social worker/Case manager contacted about plans for after hospital?
Anticipated date to leave ICU _____ and hospital _____?

What am I doing for self-care for today?

Date: _____ ICU Day #: _____

The patient's goals of care are (confirm with medical team):

Who is the medical team?

ICU Personnel	Name	Caring for Patient Until When?
Attending		
Resident/NP/PA		
Day Nurse		
Night Nurse		

Current issues (ask the ICU team for a list):

Plan for the day for each issue:

What needs to be followed up later and when is it scheduled?
   Schedule time for updates, visiting, video call?
   Labs/Tests/Procedures/Surgery?

Goals of the day:
   Spontaneous Awakening Trial?
   Spontaneous Breathing Trial?
   Physical therapist/occupational therapist/speech-language pathologist?
   Prevent Post-Intensive Care Syndrome
   Exercise/Get out of bed

Questions for the team:

Plans for discharge:
   Social worker/Case manager contacted about plans for after hospital?
   Anticipated date to leave ICU _____ and hospital _____?

What am I doing for self-care for today?

Date: _____ ICU Day #: _____

The patient's goals of care are (confirm with medical team):

Who is the medical team?

ICU Personnel	Name	Caring for Patient Until When?
Attending		
Resident/NP/PA		
Day Nurse		
Night Nurse		

Current issues (ask the ICU team for a list):

Plan for the day for each issue:

What needs to be followed up later and when is it scheduled?
  Schedule time for updates, visiting, video call?
  Labs/Tests/Procedures/Surgery?

Goals of the day:
  Spontaneous Awakening Trial?
  Spontaneous Breathing Trial?
  Physical/Occupational/Speech Therapy?
  Prevent Post-Intensive Care Syndrome
  Exercise/Get out of bed

Questions for the team:

Plans for discharge:
  Social worker/Case manager contacted about plans for after hospital?
  Anticipated date to leave ICU _____ and hospital _____?

What am I doing for self-care for today?

Date: _____ ICU Day #: _____

The patient's goals of care are (confirm with medical team):

Who is the medical team?

ICU Personnel	Name	Caring for Patient Until When?
Attending		
Resident/NP/PA		
Day Nurse		
Night Nurse		

Current issues (ask the ICU team for a list):

Plan for the day for each issue:

What needs to be followed up later and when is it scheduled?
   Schedule time for updates, visiting, video call?
   Labs/Tests/Procedures/Surgery?

Goals of the day:
   Spontaneous Awakening Trial?
   Spontaneous Breathing Trial?
   Physical therapist/occupational therapist/speech-language pathologist?
   Prevent Post-Intensive Care Syndrome
   Exercise/Get out of bed

Questions for the team:

Plans for discharge:
   Social worker/Case manager contacted about plans for after hospital?
   Anticipated date to leave ICU _____ and hospital _____?

What am I doing for self-care for today?

Date: _____ ICU Day #: _____

The patient's goals of care are (confirm with medical team):

Who is the medical team?

ICU Personnel	Name	Caring for Patient Until When?
Attending		
Resident/NP/PA		
Day Nurse		
Night Nurse		

Current issues (ask the ICU team for a list):

Plan for the day for each issue:

What needs to be followed up later and when is it scheduled?
   Schedule time for updates, visiting, video call?
   Labs/Tests/Procedures/Surgery?

Goals of the day:
   Spontaneous Awakening Trial?
   Spontaneous Breathing Trial?
   Physical/Occupational/Speech Therapy?
   Prevent Post-Intensive Care Syndrome
   Exercise/Get out of bed

Questions for the team:

Plans for discharge:
   Social worker/Case manager contacted about plans for after hospital?
   Anticipated date to leave ICU _____ and hospital _____?

What am I doing for self-care for today?

Date: _____ ICU Day #: _____

The patient's goals of care are (confirm with medical team):

Who is the medical team?

ICU Personnel	Name	Caring for Patient Until When?
Attending		
Resident/NP/PA		
Day Nurse		
Night Nurse		

Current issues (ask the ICU team for a list):

Plan for the day for each issue:

What needs to be followed up later and when is it scheduled?
    Schedule time for updates, visiting, video call?
    Labs/Tests/Procedures/Surgery?

Goals of the day:
    Spontaneous Awakening Trial?
    Spontaneous Breathing Trial?
    Physical therapist/occupational therapist/speech-language pathologist?
    Prevent Post-Intensive Care Syndrome
    Exercise/Get out of bed

Questions for the team:

Plans for discharge:
    Social worker/Case manager contacted about plans for after hospital?
    Anticipated date to leave ICU _____ and hospital _____?

What am I doing for self-care for today?

Date: _____ ICU Day #: _____

The patient's goals of care are (confirm with medical team):

Who is the medical team?

ICU Personnel	Name	Caring for Patient Until When?
Attending		
Resident/NP/PA		
Day Nurse		
Night Nurse		

Current issues (ask the ICU team for a list):

Plan for the day for each issue:

What needs to be followed up later and when is it scheduled?
   Schedule time for updates, visiting, video call?
   Labs/Tests/Procedures/Surgery?

Goals of the day:
   Spontaneous Awakening Trial?
   Spontaneous Breathing Trial?
   Physical/Occupational/Speech Therapy?
   Prevent Post-Intensive Care Syndrome
   Exercise/Get out of bed

Questions for the team:

Plans for discharge:
   Social worker/Case manager contacted about plans for after hospital?
   Anticipated date to leave ICU _____ and hospital _____?

What am I doing for self-care for today?

Date: _____ ICU Day #: _____

The patient's goals of care are (confirm with medical team):

Who is the medical team?

ICU Personnel	Name	Caring for Patient Until When?
Attending		
Resident/NP/PA		
Day Nurse		
Night Nurse		

Current issues (ask the ICU team for a list):

Plan for the day for each issue:

What needs to be followed up later and when is it scheduled?
    Schedule time for updates, visiting, video call?
    Labs/Tests/Procedures/Surgery?

Goals of the day:
    Spontaneous Awakening Trial?
    Spontaneous Breathing Trial?
    Physical therapist/occupational therapist/speech-language pathologist?
    Prevent Post-Intensive Care Syndrome
    Exercise/Get out of bed

Questions for the team:

Plans for discharge:
    Social worker/Case manager contacted about plans for after hospital?
    Anticipated date to leave ICU _____ and hospital _____?

What am I doing for self-care for today?

APPENDIX 2 Journal Outline

Use this as a quick and easy way to begin journaling. Try to add details to each section, even if it is just one or two words. This can help today and after the hospitalization.

Date: _____ ICU Day #: _____

What happened today:

Best part of the day:

Most challonging part of the day:

Questions:

Updates from friends and family:

Things to take care of outside of the hospital (people, plants, pets, mail):

Thoughts from the staff:

Pictures (if allowed)

Date: _____ ICU Day #: _____

What happened today:

Best part of the day:

Most challenging part of the day:

Questions:

Updates from friends and family:

Things to take care of outside of the hospital (people, plants, pets, mail):

Thoughts from the staff:

Pictures (if allowed)

Date: _____ ICU Day #: _____

What happened today:

Best part of the day:

Most challenging part of the day:

Questions:

Updates from friends and family:

Things to take care of outside of the hospital (people, plants, pets, mail):

Thoughts from the staff:

Pictures (if allowed)

Date: _____ ICU Day #: _____

What happened today:

Best part of the day:

Most challenging part of the day:

Questions:

Updates from friends and family:

Things to take care of outside of the hospital (people, plants, pets, mail):

Thoughts from the staff:

Pictures (if allowed)

Date: _____ ICU Day #: _____

What happened today:

Best part of the day:

Most challenging part of the day:

Questions:

Updates from friends and family:

Things to take care of outside of the hospital (people, plants, pets, mail):

Thoughts from the staff:

Pictures (if allowed)

Date: _____ ICU Day #: _____

What happened today:

Best part of the day:

Most challenging part of the day:

Questions:

Updates from friends and family:

Things to take care of outside of the hospital (people, plants, pets, mail):

Thoughts from the staff:

Pictures (if allowed)

Date: _____ ICU Day #: _____

What happened today:

Best part of the day:

Most challenging part of the day:

Questions:

Updates from friends and family:

Things to take care of outside of the hospital (people, plants, pets, mail):

Thoughts from the staff:

Pictures (if allowed)

APPENDIX 3 Get to Know Me Board

Use this as a guide to make a "get to know me board." Or, fill it out, tear it from the book, and put it up in the room. Please ask the medical staff if there is a good place for it.

Name:

Please call me:

Occupation:

My favorite
- Activities:
- Movies:
- Music:
- Books:
- Food:
- Places:

I use (glasses, hearing aids, dentures, other aids):

Things that are important to me:

What makes me proud:

Things that cheer me up:

Ways to comfort me:

What makes me stressed:

Other things I'd like you to know about me:

Photos

APPENDIX 4 Questions to Ask When Making a Decision About Care

Use these questions as a guide when making medical decisions. It is most helpful for situations when there is no clear answer. This works best when discussed with the medical team and important decision makers within the family. Questions in **bold** are most important.

- What problem occurred and in what part of the body?

- What has already been done to help the problem?

- Is more information needed (labs, tests, imaging, etc)?

- **Why is medical help needed?**

- **What are the options for treatment that align with the patient's goals of care? (Procedure vs medicine vs wait and see vs combination)**

- For each option:

  - **What is the most likely outcome for similar patients?**

  - **What is the best-case scenario and how common is it?**

  - **What is the worst-case scenario and how common is it?**

  - **How is the patient recovery and family experience in the short- and long-term?**

  - How often do the risks happen during and after?

- What do both the patient and family need to think about moving forward?

- **When does a decision need to be made?**

Figure Credits

Figure 3.1 Orbaugh SL, Gigeleisen PE. Chapter 11, Figure 1. In: *Atlas of Airway Management: Techniques and Tools*. 2nd ed. Lippincott, Williams & Wilkins; 2012.

Figure 3.2 Reprinted from Rickard CM, Marsh N, Webster J, et al. Dressings and securements for the prevention of peripheral intravenous catheter failure in adults (SAVE): a pragmatic, randomised controlled, Superiority Trial. *Lancet*. 2018;392(10145):419-430. doi:10.1016/s0140-6736(18)31380-1, with permission from Elsevier.

Figure 3.3 Reprinted from Nas MY, Ibiebele J, Dolgin G, et al. The intersection of hand hygiene, Infusion Pump Contamination, and high alarm volume in the Health Care Environment. *Am J Infect Control*. 2020;48(11):1311-1314. doi:10.1016/j.ajic.2020.04.006, with permission from Elsevier.

Figure 3.4 Guimaraes E, Davis M, Kirsch JR, Woodworth G. Chapter 4, Figure 4. In: *The Anesthesia Technologist's Manual*. 2nd ed. Lippincott, Williams & Wilkins; 2018.

Figure 4.2 Andersen FD, Degn KB, Riis Rasmussen T. Electromagnetic navigation bronchoscopy for lung nodule evaluation. patient selection, diagnostic variables and safety. *Clin Respir J*. 2020;14(6):557-563. doi:10.1111/crj.13168. © 2020 John Wiley & Sons Ltd.

Figure 4.3 Reprinted with permission from Garcilazo NHH, Hassanein M, Vachharajani TJ, Anvari E. Can I place a peripherally inserted central catheter in my patient with chronic kidney disease? *Cleve Clin J Med*. 2021;88(8):431-433. doi:10.3949/ccjm.88a.20173. Copyright © 2021 Cleveland Clinic Foundation. All rights reserved.

Figure 4.4 Ahmad H, Perez F, Rosenthal RJ. Internal jugular vein central line placement with and without ultrasound. In: Rosenthal R, Rosales A, Lo Menzo E, Dip F, eds. *Mental Conditioning to Perform Common Operations in General Surgery Training*. Springer; 2020:123-126. doi:10.1007/978-3-319-91164-9_26

Figure 4.5 Morton PG, Fontaine DK. Chapter 16, Figure 2. In: *Essentials of Critical Care Nursing: A Holistic Approach*. 1st ed. Lippincott, Williams & Wilkins; 2012.

Morton PG, Fontaine DK. Chapter 25, Figure 4. In: *Critical Care Nursing: A Holistic Approach*. 1st ed. Lippincott, Williams & Wilkins; 2017.

Figure 4.6 https://www.cancer.gov/publications/dictionaries/cancer-terms/def/upper-endoscopy

Winslow T. *Upper Endoscopy*. 2005. Accessed February 19, 2022. https://www.teresewinslow.com/#/digestion/. © 2005 Terese Winslow LLC, U.S. Govt. has certain rights.

Figure 4.8 Republished with permission of MA Healthcare Limited, from Palmer SJ. An overview of enteral feeding in the community. *Br J Community Nurs*. 2021;26(1):26-29. doi:10.12968/bjcn.2021.26.1.26, permission conveyed through Copyright Clearance Center, Inc.

Figure 4.9 Reprinted with permission from Garcilazo NH, Hassanein M, Vachharajani TJ, Anvari E. Can I place a peripherally inserted central catheter in my patient with chronic kidney disease? *Cleve Clin J Med*. 2021;88(8):431-433. doi:10.3949/ccjm.88a.20173. Copyright © 2021 Cleveland Clinic Foundation. All rights reserved.

Figure 4.10 From *Hemodynamic Monitoring Made Incredibly Visual*. 2nd ed. Lippincott, Williams & Wilkins; 2010.

Figure 4.11 National Heart, Lung, and Blood Institute; National Institutes of Health; U.S. Department of Health and Human Services.

Figure 4.12 Carter PJ, Goldschmidt WM. Chapter 26, Figure 6. In: Rosenthal R, Rosales A, Lo Menzo E, Dip F, eds. *Lippincott's Textbook for Long-Term Care Nursing Assistants: A Humanistic Approach to Health Care*. 1st ed. Lippincott, Williams & Wilkins; 2009.

Figure 5.2 BIS JPN by ignis is licensed under the Creative Commons Attribution-Share Alike 3.0 Unported license.

Figure 5.3 Hickey JV. Chapter 8, Figure 9. In: *The Clinical Practice of Neurological and Neurosurgical Nursing*. 8th ed. Lippincott, Williams & Wilkins, 2019.

Figure 7.1 Frendl G, Urman RD. Chapter 5, Figure 4. In: *Pocket ICU*. 2nd ed. Lippincott, Williams & Wilkins; 2017.

Figure 7.2 Carter PJ, Goldschmidt WM. Chapter 18, Figure 7d. In: *Lippincott's Textbook for Long-Term Care Nursing Assistants: A Humanistic Approach to Health Care*. 1st ed. Lippincott, Williams & Wilkins; 2009.

Figure 7.3 Carter PJ. Chapter 10, Figure 5c. In: *Lippincott's Textbook for Nursing Assistants: A Humanistic Approach to Caregiving*. 3rd ed. Lippincott, Williams & Wilkins; 2011.

Figure 7.4 Chung KC, van Aalst J, Mehrara B, Disa JJ, Lee G, Gosain A. Part 4, Chapter 17, Figure 2. In: *Flaps in Plastic and Reconstructive Surgery*. Lippincott, Williams & Wilkins; 2019.

Figure 7.5 Taylor C, Lynn P, Bartlett JL. Chapter 32, Figure 4. In: *Fundamentals of Nursing: The Art and Science of Person-Centered Care*. 9th ed. Lippincott, Williams & Wilkins; 2018.

Figure 8.1 Carter PJ. Chapter 33, Figure 8a. In: *Lippincott's Textbook for Nursing Assistants: A Humanistic Approach to Caregiving*. 3rd ed. Lippincott, Williams & Wilkins; 2011.

Figure 8.2 Macedo E, Cerdá J. Choosing a CRRT machine and modality. *Semin Dial*. 2021;34(6):423-431. doi:10.1111/sdi.13029. © 2021 Wiley Periodicals LLC.

Figure 8.3 Nasal Cannula (Adult) by BruceBlaus is licensed under Creative Commons Attribution-Share Alike 4.0 International license.

Figure 8.4 Springhouse. Chapter 6, Figure 15b. In: *Nursing Procedures Made Incredibly Easy!* 1st ed. Wolters Kluwer Health; 2001.

Figure 8.5 This article/chapter was published in Göksu E, Kılıç D, İbze S. Non-invasive ventilation in the ED: Whom, when, how? *Turk J Emerg Med*. 2018;18(2):52-56. doi:10.1016/j.tjem.2018.01.002, Copyright Elsevier (2018).

Springhouse. *Lippincott's Visual Encyclopedia of Clinical Skills*. Wolters Kluwer Health; 2009.

Figure 8.6 Marini JJ, Drics DJ. Chapter 7, Figure 12. In: *Critical Care Medicine: The Essentials and More*. 5th ed. Lippincott, Williams & Wilkins; 2018.

Figure 8.7 Republished with permission of Daedalus Enterprises Inc, from Kacmarek RM. The mechanical ventilator: Past, present, and future. *Respir Care*. American Association for Inhalation Therapy; American Association for Respiratory Therapy; American Association for Respiratory Care. 2011;56(8):1170-1180. doi:10.4187/respcare.01420, permission conveyed through Copyright Clearance Center, Inc.

Figure 8.8 Guimaraes E, Davis M, Kirsch JR, Woodworth G. Chapter 18, Figure 3. In: *The Anesthesia Technologist's Manual*. 2nd ed. Lippincott, Williams & Wilkins; 2018.

Figure 8.9 Carter PJ. Chapter 6, Figure 7. In: *Lippincott Acute Care Skills for Advanced Nursing Assistants: A Humanistic Approach to Caregiving.* 1st ed. Lippincott, Williams & Wilkins; 2019.

Figure 9.2 Herzog E. Chapter 28, Figure 2. In: *Cardiac Care Unit Survival Guide.* Lippincott, Williams & Wilkins; 2012.

Lippincott Williams and Wilkins, *Pathophysiology Made Incredibly Visual.* 3rd ed. Lippincott Williams & Wilkins; 2016.

Capriotti T. Chapter 2, Figure DVT. In: *Pathophysiology Made Incredibly Visual!* 3rd ed. Lippincott, Williams & Wilkins; 2016.

Figure 9.3 Timby BK, Smith NE. Chapter 38, Figure 3. In: *Introductory Medical-Surgical Nursing.* 12th ed. Lippincott, Williams & Wilkins; 2017.

Figure 13.1 Guimaraes E, Woodworth G, Davis M, Kirsch JR. Chapter 11, Figure 7. In: *The Anesthesia Technologists Manual.* 2nd ed. Lippincott, Williams & Wilkins; 2018.

Index

Note: Page numbers followed by 'f' indicate figures.

Psychiatry on the Stage